ADHD is Not an Illness and Ritalin is Not a Cure

A Comprehensive Rebuttal of the (alleged) Scientific Consensus

ADHD is Not an Illness and Ritalin is Not a Cure

A Comprehensive Rebuttal of the (alleged) Scientific Consensus

Yaakov Ophir, PhD

Technion - Israel Institute of Technology, Israel

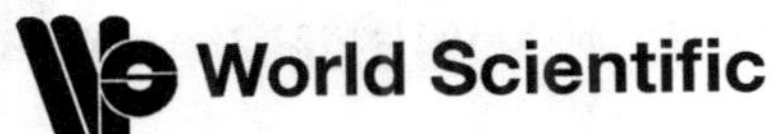

NEW JERSEY • LONDON • SINGAPORE • BEIJING • SHANGHAI • HONG KONG • TAIPEI • CHENNAI • TOKYO

Published by

World Scientific Publishing Co. Pte. Ltd.
5 Toh Tuck Link, Singapore 596224
USA office: 27 Warren Street, Suite 401-402, Hackensack, NJ 07601
UK office: 57 Shelton Street, Covent Garden, London WC2H 9HE

Library of Congress Cataloging-in-Publication Data
Names: Ophir, Yaakov, author.
Title: ADHD is not an illness and ritalin is not a cure : a comprehensive rebuttal of the (alleged) scientific consensus / Yaakov Ophir, Technion - Israel Institute of Technology, Israel.
Description: Hackensack, NJ : World Scientific, [2022] | Includes bibliographical references and index.
Identifiers: LCCN 2022004980 | ISBN 9789811253225 (hardcover) | ISBN 9789811254130 (paperback) | ISBN 9789811253232 (ebook for institutions) | ISBN 9789811253249 (ebook for individuals)
Subjects: LCSH: Attention-deficit hyperactivity disorder. | Methylphenidate.
Classification: LCC RJ506.H9 O64 2022 | DDC 618.92/8589--dc23/eng/20220318
LC record available at https://lccn.loc.gov/2022004980

British Library Cataloguing-in-Publication Data
A catalogue record for this book is available from the British Library.

First published 2022 (hardcover)
Reprinted 2023 (in paperback edition)
ISBN 978-981-125-413-0 (pbk)

Disclaimer: The author acknowledges the controversy about Attention Deficit Hyperactivity Disorder (ADHD) and its associated pharmacological treatments and declares that the content of the book reflects his own view as a scientist practitioner. The scientific rebuttal brought in this book should not be interpreted as a concrete and personal medical advice. Any practical decisions should be made cautiously, under proper medical supervision, especially if they involve medications (reducing medications can be a tough, lengthy, and even dangerous process). Bearing this cautionary disclaimer in mind, the author wishes to upraise another principal ethical rule in medicine, which is the universally accepted norm of *informed consent*. In his view, scientists and practitioners are obligated to provide the public with transparent, wide-scope, and credible information, even if this information does not align with the (alleged) consensus. This is the only way, in his view, parents could really be given the freedom to choose the best clinical/educational roads for their children, especially considering the fact that these roads are diverged, controversial, and sometimes masked by a thick smoke of conflicts of interests.

For any available supplementary material, please visit
https://www.worldscientific.com/worldscibooks/10.1142/12752#t=suppl

To Maayan,
My very special flamingo

Personal Prologue
A late apology to Queen Sarabi

"Ritalin will help your son stop feeling dumb," I tried to persuade her for the 100th time, but she, with the sharp intuition that only brave mothers like her have, was not convinced. "You are wrong," she said confidently (let's call her Queen Sarabi), despite the fact that over ten years ago, I was on the 'right' side of the debate over Attention Deficit Hyperactivity Disorder (ADHD), and despite the fact that the entire galactic empire backed me up in my sacred mission: the teachers, the school director, the doctors, and above all, the scientists. Queen Sarabi, in contrast, took her stand against our droid army alone, without money and without education. "My son is perfect exactly as he is," she said. "He's not sick. Nothing is wrong with his brain, and he doesn't have any H-D-H-D or whatever you therapists call this lifelong medical condition."

As a young psychologist, I was not deterred. I decided to operate our heavy psychological weapon and target her innate parental worries: "Your son (let's call him Simba), is accumulating multiple discouraging experiences," I argued beautifully, like a well-trained litigator. "His self-esteem is continuously under attack. If he is not treated with medications, he will grow up feeling excessive guilt for all his misbehaviors." "Well," she roared quietly, "so maybe it's time to stop blaming my child's personality for everything. He is not evil. Someone else is (let's call this "someone" Scar)." At the end of the story, a medical miracle occurred. Simba was healed. His terrible lifelong illness disappeared. His lioness-mother simply transferred him to a different, more inclusive school, in which the teachers managed to see the child as a whole, beyond his specific difficulties. Like Queen Sarabi, the adult caregivers in this new school believed that Simba could become "a mighty king" one day ("so enemies beware"), if he is only given the proper psycho-educational chance.

I stood firm. I would not let any miracle shake my beliefs, let alone bring me to apologize to 'uneducated' mothers who did not go to a prestigious university, like I did. After all, I knew that ADHD is a genuine biomedical condition that is inscribed in the Bible — our holy *Diagnostic and Statistical Manual of Mental Disorders* (*DSM*). Only several years later, when my own first-born child was diagnosed (at the unbelievable age of 4 years!), I began to reconsider my original, consensual position regarding ADHD.

I realize that this last personal fact (which implies that I am emotionally involved in the topic at hand) might be used against me as an excuse not to consider the substantiative arguments that will be brought forth in this book. That's fine. I respect this position, though this personal investment cannot be compared to the massive conflicts of interests that characterize much of the 'consensual' research on ADHD (see Chapter 12). I also forgive my opponents, in advance, for their expected argumentum ad hominem insults. I admit that, when I first voiced my 'heretical' position regarding ADHD (in Hebrew), I was shocked, and a bit shaken, by the intensity of the aggressive academic and medical response. Alongside dozens of encouraging phone calls and tear-soaked letters from suffering parents who suddenly felt understood, I received numerous hostile internet-prescriptions (of at least 100 milligrams each) filled with angry accusations that scared me. "The author [me] is an ignorant person," they said. "The author is a dangerous person," they said, not forgetting to remind me of my greatest sin: "The author is not a Medical Doctor."

Today, however, I plead guilty with honor. I am not a Doctor of Medicine (M.D). I am 'just' a Doctor of Philosophy (PhD) who conducts scientific research on psychopathology (mainly in the context of the digital age) and teaches basic research methodologies and critical thinking. Although I believe that this book should not be judged by its author's cover (i.e., academic and professional titles), I recognize people's need for a 'white coat' authority so here is mine: I am a research associate at the Technion — Israel Institute of Technology and I am a licensed clinical psychologist with specific expertise in child and adolescent psychology. In this context, I have gathered large clinical, real-life experience with 'ADHD children' as well as with their courageous mothers and fathers. The lasts are in fact, the real addressees of this book. Although this book is written to fellow scientists, in somewhat formal academic language, with hundreds of scientific references and dozens of statistical computations, I address this book to my fellow parents, who were surprised to learn, like I was, that their healthy and happy boy or girl was born with a lifelong neurodevelopmental disorder that, if left untreated with psychoactive drugs, could deteriorate, and cause pervasive damage. For these coping parents, I decided to embark on this career-risking journey, in which I am trying to uncover and organize the somewhat hidden science behind ADHD and stimulant medications (the first-line pharmacological treatment for ADHD). I know I am about ten years late, but I ask for your forgiveness, wise lioness mother. Please accept this book as a late peace offering.

Of course, I am not traveling this rocky road alone. I drive a powerful off-road jeep that was built by scientific giants (see the following Introduction Chapter). However, I am aware of the sensitivity of the debate over ADHD, and I promise to approach it from a clean and modest position, while anchoring every argument on pure logic and solid scientific evidence. Aside from these opening remarks and the personal closing statements at the end of the book (Personal Epilogue), everything that you are about to read in this book is written in a rigid and careful manner, mostly in line with standard academic style. Yes, I use metaphors and sometimes more casual language to ease the reading, but I adhere to conventional scientific norms. I have also asked Prof. Richard Silberstein, a well-acknowledged cognitive neuroscientist (who had actually done research that yielded brain differences between ADHD and non-ADHD populations), to conduct a rigorous scientific review of the book. I truly hope that the reader will adopt the same approach and dare to ask honestly: Perhaps the galactic empire's perception about ADHD is inaccurate?

Although I am not a Medical Doctor, I too believe that we should "first, do no harm" and adhere to core medical ethics that require us to provide our patients with clear and transparent information regarding the historical debate

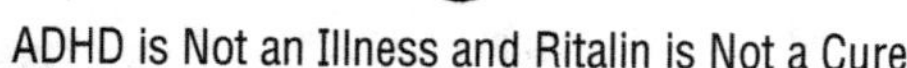

over the validity of ADHD and the legitimacy of its first-line treatments with psychostimulants. I therefore invite whoever is willing to engage in a piercing, yet evidence-based, scientific discourse, to dive into the deep scientific literature with me, and explore the underlying questions of this book: Do millions of children really suffer from a genuine neuropsychiatric disorder called ADHD? Is it really such a good idea to treat all these children with powerful psychoactive medications? If you have even the slightest worry that the answer to both questions is simply 'no,' then you must read this book.

Yours,
Yaakov

Contents

“

“ADHD is the diabetes of psychiatry, it's a chronic disorder that has to be managed every day to prevent the secondary harms it's going to cause, but there is no cure for this disorder.”

Barkley, R. A. (2012). Keynote lecture at the 2012 Burnett Seminar for Academic Achievement [1]

Introduction
Illusory consensus and silenced controversy

Is Attention Deficit Hyperactivity Disorder (ADHD) a valid medical condition? Allegedly, the answer to this question is simple (and why bother writing a whole book about it?). According to the International Consensus Statement, published by a large consortium of experts led by Prof. Russell Barkley, there is "overwhelming" evidence that ADHD is a genuine and dangerous disorder with traceable bioneurological markers and genetic foundations [2]. ADHD, the most prevalent neuropsychiatric label in children [3, 4], is repeatedly depicted by leaders of the field as an objective and chronic medical condition that should be managed regularly, preferably with stimulant medications [2, 5–8]. But what if they are all wrong? What if ADHD does not meet the required criteria for a neuropsychiatric disorder? Is it possible that millions of children are being labeled and treated unjustifiably, with powerful and highly dangerous psychoactive drugs?

The book that you are about to read is dedicated to the investigation of these very questions, but first we need to fully understand the somewhat deterministic biomedical position of the presumed scientific consensus. In one of the previous incarnations of ADHD, the disorder was called Minimal Brain Damage [9] and many physicians, including influential figures such as Prof. Joseph Biederman from Harvard Medical School still refer to ADHD as a chronic "brain disorder" [10, p. 1239]. Correspondingly, the *Diagnostic and Statistical Manual of Mental Disorders* (*DSM*)[1] — perhaps the most influential psychiatric authority — places ADHD within the manual section on neurodevelopmental disorders, right after Intellectual Disabilities and Autism

---

1 Unless written otherwise, all references to the Diagnostic and Statistical Manual of Mental Disorders (DSM) in this book pertain to the 5th edition of the manual (i.e., DSM-5) that was published by the American Psychiatric Association (APA) in 2013. It is noted that a text revision of this edition was published in March 2022 (DSM-5-TR), during the production process of this book, however no substantial changes in the diagnosis of ADHD were declared by the APA.

Spectrum Disorder [4]. A recent European consensus statement even extends this mainly childhood disorder to "a neurodevelopmental and heritable disorder with a lifespan perspective: starting in childhood, persisting in adulthood until old age, with significant psycho-social impairment, a high comorbidity rate and multimorbidity" [6, p. 27]. Inevitably, this biomedical view, as if human behaviors can be explained purely by biogenetic factors, leads to biochemical solutions (with or without other, non-medical accommodations). Psychostimulant medications, such as methylphenidate (e.g., Ritalin) and amphetamines (e.g., Adderall), are prescribed in unprecedented amounts to the majority of the children diagnosed with the disorder [11, 12] and are considered the pharmacological *treatment of choice* for ADHD [8, 13–15].

The diagnostic clinical picture

So how does this lifelong brain disorder manifest in children's daily lives? Aside from a plain difficulty to sustain attention for prolonged durations, children with ADHD are claimed to have poor *cognitive control* [16] — an ingrained deficit in the brain's *executive functions*, which are the set of cognitive abilities that allow us to control and regulate our behaviors and responses. Leading theories emphasize the relatively poor ability of children with ADHD to engage in *cognitive inhibition* — a crucial executive function that allows us to resist, or tune out, internal thoughts and external stimuli that are irrelevant to us at a given task [16, 17]. From a real-life, clinical point of view, this cognitive impairment is manifested, according to the current edition of the *DSM*, in two clusters of symptoms — a cluster that is termed *inattention*, and a cluster that is termed *hyperactivity and impulsivity*. Each cluster includes nine potential symptoms, and the diagnostic criteria require that at least six symptoms of one of these clusters be evident. Representative symptoms of inattention are: "often fails to give close attention to details or makes careless mistakes in schoolwork, at work, or during other activities," "often has difficulty sustaining attention in tasks or play activities," and "often has difficulty organizing tasks and activities". Representative symptoms of hyperactivity and impulsivity are: "often fidgets with or taps hands or feet or squirms in seat," "often leaves seat in situations when remaining seated is expected," and "often runs about or climbs in situations where it is inappropriate" [18, pp. 59–60].

Indeed, to an outside viewer, these official symptoms of ADHD may seem like common and somewhat benign behaviors of many children, but make no mistake, according to the abovementioned consortium of scientists, these behaviors, and the assumed neuropsychological impairments that underlie them, "can cause devastating problems" and "pose serious harm to most individuals possessing the disorder" [2, pp. 89–90]. Science has determined, according to representatives of the consensus, that ADHD has adverse implications for almost every life domain [19] and that it involves "serious economic implications for children, families, and society" [6, p. 25]. Although such a deterministic biomedical view of mental disorders is less common in general psychiatry today than it used to be in the past [20, 21], the biomedical paradigm still rules the clinical field of ADHD.

To get the essence of the biomedical view, it is worth listening to the recorded keynote lecture by Barkley, which was mentioned above. To my knowledge, Prof. Barkley is considered the leading authority in ADHD today and his words seem to represent the mainstream and widely accepted beliefs about the disorder. Here is a small part of this influential lecture:

> "You have a brain; the back part is where you learn, and the front part is where you do... ADHD splits them apart... You can be the brightest kid in the world, not gonna matter. So you have a real problem on your hands... it interferes with all seven executive functions... what does this means for treatment? Teaching skills is inadequate. It won't work... all of this in ADHD is due to neurogenetic deficits and that means that medications are absolutely justifiable. After all, if you have a neurogenetic disorder, then neurogenetic therapies have a role to play in the disorder. And they do. 80% of people with ADHD will be on medications for some point in their life. And it's a good thing. It's the most effective thing

we have. There are other things we can do but this is the most effective... It means that ADHD is the diabetes of psychiatry, it's a chronic disorder that has to be managed every day to prevent the secondary harms it's going to cause, but there is no cure for this disorder. Now, about 1 in 6 people might outgrow it, maybe it's 1 in 3, we're not sure yet, but the vast majority, two thirds will continue to have ADHD in adulthood, and they need to view ADHD as the diabetes of the brain. It's a chronic disorder" [1].

The intense and longstanding debate

But how consensual is the biomedical view about ADHD articulated in this straightforward keynote lecture? According to Barkley's 2002 International Consensus Statement, the answer to this question is clear: "As a matter of science, the notion that ADHD does not exist is simply wrong... All of the major medical associations and government health agencies recognize ADHD as a genuine disorder" [2, p. 89]. In fact, this consensus statement is packed with conclusive and combative remarks that dismiss and diminish any other perspective on this subject: "The views of **a handful of nonexpert doctors** that ADHD does not exist are contrasted against mainstream scientific views... Such attempts at balance give the public the impression that there is substantial scientific disagreement over whether ADHD is a real medical condition. In fact, **there is no such disagreement**... As attested to by the numerous scientists signing this document, **there is no question**... that ADHD involves a serious deficiency... and **there is no doubt** that ADHD leads to impairments... To publish **stories** that ADHD is a fictitious disorder... is tantamount to declaring **the earth flat, the laws of gravity debatable, and the periodic table in chemistry a fraud**" (bold added by Y.O.).

The debate within the Consensus Development Conference

And yet, despite these harsh statements, the very conference that was set by the US National Institute of Mental Health (NIMH) to formulate a consensual perception regarding the diagnosis and treatment of ADHD, only a few years earlier, drew a more nuanced picture. The document that summarized the conference opened with plain statements that "some persons have suggested that ADHD is just normal childhood behavior" and that "despite the substantial progress… the disorder has remained controversial in many public and private sectors" [13, p. 1]. Specifically, a major point of dispute, according to this document, concerns the legitimacy of psychostimulants as a leading treatment for ADHD. Indeed, most of the participants of this conference seemed to accept the term ADHD as a useful label to depict children's difficulties. However, the emerging picture of their various approaches is not one-dimensional.

For example, the opening overview of the disorder by Dr. Keith Conners — one of the founders of the field who is sometimes referred to as the 'father of ADHD' — warns of "serious underdiagnosis or overdiagnosis, resulting in excesses or deficiencies of pharmacologic treatments" [13, p. 23]. Moreover, in this overview, Conners had actually challenged the neurological foundation of the disorder arguing that the neuroimaging studies reflect "a poor understanding of any specificity for the neural basis of ADHD". Finally, he dared to raise questions regarding the very validity of the diagnosis when he said: "The high levels of comorbidity… also call into question the specificity of the definition of the disease and whether current criteria are sufficient to allow further understanding of the neurobiology of the syndrome" (p. 23). Needless to say that over a decade later, Dr. Conners has amazed the scientific community with his declaration that the rates of ADHD reflect "a national disaster of dangerous proportions" (see also Chapter 2). "The numbers make it look like an epidemic," he said, "well, it's not. It's preposterous. This is a concoction to justify the giving out of medication at unprecedented and unjustifiable levels" [22].

Importantly, the Consensus Development Conference also gave voice to known critics of the disorder and its treatment. For example, in a section titled "Is Attention Deficit Hyperactivity Disorder a Valid Disorder?", Dr. William Carey, an admired clinician and researcher from the School of Medicine at

UPenn (i.e., not a "nonexpert doctor" who believes that the "earth is flat"), listed several crucial problems in the diagnostic terminology of ADHD. This list includes brief descriptions of some core problems that are discussed in length in the current book, such as: the lack of clear evidence for brain dysregulations, the dismissal of environmental factors, and the absence of reasonable evolutionary perspective [23, 24]. In Carey's view, "what is now most often described as ADHD… appears to be a set of normal behavioral variations that sometimes lead to dysfunction through dissonant environmental interactions. This discrepancy leaves the validity of the construct in doubt" [13, p. 35].

Similarly, psychiatrist Dr. Peter Breggin, a well-known critic of psychiatric treatments, had presented in this Consensus Development Conference a long list of adverse outcomes that associate with the pharmacological treatment of choice for ADHD. Dr. Breggin had later published numerous articles and books that challenged the legitimacy of psychiatric drugs, including designated books about ADHD, such as "the Ritalin fact book: What your doctor won't tell you about ADHD and stimulant drugs" [25]. Indeed, Dr. Breggin has been labeled by many as a rebel against mainstream psychiatry, but other more conventional scholars have also raised serious concerns regarding the treatment of choice for ADHD. Prof. Nadine Lambert from UC Berkeley, for example, reported evidence from a prospective longitudinal study, which suggested that the use of ADHD medications in childhood is associated with smoking and drug abuse (mainly cocaine) in adulthood [26].

Finally, several contributors of the Consensus Development Conference, such as Prof. James Swanson, who presented favorable views regarding the neurological foundation of ADHD, and Prof. Peter Jensen who reviewed the benefits of careful medication treatments, had later articulated severe reservations regarding their initial stance following their seminal longitudinal research on the topic (Chapter 9). Jensen reported that stimulant medications are not effective in the long term and that they can actually worsen the person's symptoms [27], and Swanson had even represented the "against" position in a recent debate regarding the long-term efficacy of stimulant medications [28].

In the meantime, it also turned out that influential proponents of the disorder from the Consensus Development Conference failed to declare their relationships with the pharma industry,[2] in which they received at least US$1.6 million in consulting fees [29, 30].

The extensive historical debate

Of course, the controversy does not stop within the borders of the Consensus Development Conference. Together with 33 co-endorsers, the influential British psychiatrist, Prof. Sami Timimi from the University of Lincoln published a seminal critique of Barkley's consensus statement, whereby he challenged the biological deterministic view of ADHD and proposed a more integrative cultural perspective [31]. In fact, Timimi and his co-authors had challenged the very act of formulating a conclusive consensus statement. "Not only is it completely counter to the spirit and practice of science to cease questioning the validity of ADHD… there is an ethical and moral responsibility to do so" [31, p. 59]. Instead of encouraging healthy scientific debates, such dogmatic consensual statements silence opponents and suppress all contradictory information that could lead to desirable development in the existing medical paradigm [32]. Fortunately, Timimi did not surrender to this bullying act and continued to publish numerous articles and books, in which he argued that ADHD is a troubling illustration of poor medicine, and that we should shift our perspective of children's behaviors from brain deficits to cultural and sociological frameworks [e.g., 33, 34, 35].

And Prof. Timimi is not alone. Table 1 presents only a partial list of excellent critical articles and books about ADHD and stimulant medications, which were written by recognized experts who are by no means "gravity deniers". The perspectives of these critiques vary from pure biology and medicine to wider perspectives that integrate sociology, anthropology, economics, and even history, but essentially, they all question the validity of what they sometimes call the

---

2 I try to avoid mentioning actual names of researchers who failed to report of conflicts of interests because my purpose here is not to discredit anyone specific, but to expose the more general problem of poor reliability.

Table 1. Partial list of critical articles and books about ADHD and stimulant medications (organized alphabetically)

Author(s)	**Affiliation**	**Critical book/article**
Antonio Maturo	University of Bologna	The medicalization of education: ADHD, human enhancement and academic performance (2013)
Blake Harding	Independent scholar	The Field Guide to ADHD: What They Don't Want You to Know (2017)
Dale Archer	The Institute for Neuropsychiatry in Lake Charles	The ADHD advantage: What you thought was a diagnosis may be your greatest strength (2015)
David Foreman	King's College London	Attention-deficit hyperactivity disorder (ADHD): progress and controversy in diagnosis and treatment (2018)
Gabor Mate	Independent scholar	Scattered Minds: A New Look at the Origins and Healing of Attention Deficit Disorder (2019)
James Swanson	University of California	Are stimulant medications for ADHD effective in the long-term? (Against) (2019)
Jeanne Stolzer	University of Nebraska at Kearney	Attention deficit hyperactivity disorder: valid medical condition or culturally constructed myth? (2009)
Jerome Kagan	Harvard University	What about tutoring instead of pills? (2012)
Jim Wilson	Greenwich Child and Adolescent Mental Health Service, London	A social relational critique of the biomedical definition and treatment of ADHD; ethical practical and political implications (2013)

Joanna Moncrieff & Sami Timimi	University College London	Is ADHD a valid diagnosis in adults? No (2010)
Johan Wiklund *et al.*	Syracuse University	ADHD, impulsivity and entrepreneurship (2017)
John Visser & Zenib Jehan	University of Birmingham	ADHD: a scientific fact or a factual opinion? A critique of the veracity of Attention Deficit Hyperactivity Disorder (2009)
Jonathan Leo	Lincoln Memorial University	American Preschoolers on Ritalin (2002)
Jonathan Leo & David Cohen	Lincoln Memorial University Florida International University	Broken brains or flawed studies? A critical review of ADHD neuroimaging research (2003)
Klaus Lange *et al.*	University of Regensburg	The history of attention deficit hyperactivity disorder (2010)
Marylin Wedge	Practitioner/Independent scholar	A Disease Called Childhood: Why ADHD Became an American Epidemic (2016)
Matthew Smith	University of Strathclyde	Hyperactive around the world? The history of ADHD in global perspective (2017)
Michael Corrigan	Independent scholar	Debunking ADHD: 10 Reasons to Stop Drugging Kids for Acting Like Kids (2014)
Peter Breggin	Center for the Study of Empathic Therapy	The Ritalin fact book: What your doctor won't tell you about ADHD and stimulant drugs (2009)
Peter Gray	Boston College	The harm of coercive schooling (2020)
Richard Saul	Highland Park Hospital	ADHD does not exist (2014)

(*Continued*)

Table 1. (*Continued*)

Author(s)	Affiliation	Critical book/article
Rick Mayes *et al.*	University of Richmond	Medicating Children: ADHD and Pediatric Mental Health (2009)
Russell Searight & Lesley McLaren	Saint Louis University	Attention-deficit hyperactivity disorder: The medicalization of misbehavior (1998)
Sami Timimi	University of Lincoln	Attention deficit hyperactivity disorder is an example of bad medicine; The social construction of attention deficit hyperactivity disorder (2015)
Sami Timimi & 33 Co-endorsers	University of Lincoln	A critique of the international consensus statement on ADHD
Stephen Hinshaw & Richard Scheffler	UC San Francisco UC Berkeley	The ADHD Explosion: Myths, Medication, Money, and Today's Push for Performance (2014)
Thom Hartmann	Independent scholar	ADHD: A hunter in a farmer's world (2019)
Thomas Armstrong	Independent scholar	The myth of the ADHD child (2017)
William Carey	University of Pennsylvania School of Medicine	Is attention deficit hyperactivity disorder a valid disorder? (1998)

'myth' of ADHD [e.g., 9, 36, 37–42]. The next chapter (Chapter 1) outlines the various types of reliability and validity that might be impaired in ADHD (Box 1), but it is important to mention here that certain validity gaps can demolish an entire theory. For example, to my understanding, based on a specific problem known as poor discriminant validity, neurologist Richard Saul had published a facinating rebuttal book under the blatant title: "ADHD Does Not Exist" [43]. In the same spirit, Harvard Professor Jerome Kagan openly called the disorder "an invention", arguing that 90% of the millions of children diagnosed with ADHD do not suffer from brain dysregulations [44].

To use a football cliché, at this stage of the introduction, it seems safe to conclude that the "table doesn't lie". The above saying according to which "there is no such disagreement" [2, p. 89] is not accurate, to say the least. The biomedical approach regarding ADHD, as illustrated above, is not so consensual as one might think. Further in this book, we will encounter many more researchers who challenged the validity of the disorder and the legitimacy of its associated medications, but even the short list of critics presented above demonstrates well why I chose to add the word 'alleged' before the term 'scientific consensus' in the title of the book. The apparent consensus regarding ADHD is an illusion driven and intensified by powerful parties of interest (see Chapter 12). The reality is that ADHD and stimulant medications stand at the heart of a vital and long-standing controversy in the medical, legal, and ethical discourse [45–47].

Not only is the debate alive, kicking, and sometimes, daring to raise its repressed head, arguments against the validity of ADHD have penetrated the mainstream (pro-ADHD) medical discourse. Multiple scholars who accept the label of ADHD are still warning against overdiagnosis and overmedication of millions of children [48, 49]. In fact, a recent study conducted among hundreds of mainstream Israeli physicians (i.e., not critics of ADHD) — specialists in children neurology, psychiatry, or development — revealed that most physicians (70.1%) believe that there has been a moderate-to-significant increase in unreliable diagnoses of ADHD [50]. More than 36% of the physicians believed that, at least 21% of children with ADHD are given the diagnosis despite an inconclusive clinical evaluation and about 5% of the physicians believed that more than 50% (!) of the ADHD diagnoses are unreliable (needless to say that the participating physicians were not provided with the updated information that will be presented in Chapter 2 regarding the extremely high prevalence of ADHD in Israel). Indeed, concerns regarding overdiagnosis are not equal to explicit critiques of the very validity of the disorder, but when the overdiagnosis rates are extremely high, there is a large overlap between the two (for a detailed explanation of this claim, see Chapter 2).

Be that as it may, whether the criticisms are anecdotal or pervasive, it seems that the last word on this burning subject has not yet been said. There is now a growing number of esteemed researchers who point to the contradictions that exist within the biomedical model, refuse to perceive ADHD as a valid medical label, and call to remove it from the medical realm [e.g., 47, 51, 52]. A representative well-articulated critique can be found in the recently updated edition of "The Myth of the ADHD Child", a founding book by Dr. Thomas Armstrong that uncovers the psycho-social and -educational (i.e., not biological) causes of ADHD and provides 101 non-pharmacological ways to improve children's attention and behaviors [53]. Like Armstrong, there are many other scholars and clinicians who oppose the alleged consensus and hold the position that normative behaviors of children (e.g., "often fails to finish schoolwork", "often runs about or climbs") are being medicalized unjustifiably, mainly in response to school-related pressure and demands [54, 55]. Overall, despite the dominance of the biomedical approach, the starting point of the present book is that ADHD is, at the very least, a controversial disorder.

The current book

Building on previous critiques (some of which are mentioned above), the current book offers a comprehensive and in-depth scientific rebuttal of the alleged consensus about ADHD and stimulant medications. Aside from gathering multiple key critiques and integrating them within one consolidated scientific source (and I apologize for not mentioning all the available critiques), this book dives deep into the major controversies over ADHD and explores the available evidence, for and against, the alleged consensus. As implied in my Personal Prologue, I have made considerable efforts to make the rough science as accessible as I can (mainly to parents), but readers should be prepared for a relatively high-resolution inspection of methodologies, statistical analyses, research findings, and writing tactics. This in-depth review of the intrinsic (and sometimes biased and corrupted) scientific details, is the only way I know to reveal the unstable foundations of the governing biomedical perception about ADHD.

Specifically, Part One of this book comprises a step-by-step refutation of the notion that ADHD is an objective and scientifically valid neuropsychiatric disorder. In this part, I first lay out the founding philosophical assumptions that are needed for the validity discussion of any psychopathology (Chapter 1), including the four conventional criteria for diagnosing abnormal behavior — the criteria of deviance, dysfunction, danger, and distress (Chapters 2-5). This part also emphasizes the importance of distinguishing severe neuropsychiatric conditions from normative, non-pathological ADHD-like behaviors (Chapter 5) and provides a detailed rebuttal of the proclaimed biogenetic nature of ADHD (Chapter 6). By thoroughly discussing each criterion, Part One exposes numerous methodological failures and peculiar attributes of ADHD that shake the validity foundations of ADHD (see also Table 4 at the General Discussion section) and show that ADHD cannot be categorized as an objective brain deficit or as a psychiatric disorder (see also the Interim Summary of Part One).

Part Two refutes the notion that stimulant medications should be considered as a legitimate and desirable treatment. After a short introductory of stimulant medications and their unprecedented prescription rates (Chapter 7), this part rigorously reviews dozens of widely accepted scientific sources (comprehensive literature reviews, meta-analysis studies, longitudinal studies, randomized controlled studies, and clinical case studies) that addressed the short-term efficacy (Chapter 8) and the long-term efficacy (Chapter 9) of stimulant medications, as well as their 'non-serious' side-effects (Chapter 10) and highly serious and long-term adverse outcomes (Chapter 11). Part Two also discusses the dangerous operative mechanism of stimulant medications (Chapter 11) and shows that, altogether, the clinical value of these drugs is highly limited. Not only are the medications not effective in the long run, prolonged usage can also trigger ADHD-like symptoms and lead to long-term biochemical dysregulations and sustainable physical and mental damage (see also the Interim Summary of Part Two). In Part Two, I also discuss the numerous distortions — scientific biases and misconducts — that occur in the biomedical research on ADHD and its related medications and uncover the forces that stand behind the alleged consensus — forces with large economic interests that might explain how it is the case that the public is unaware of the massive evidence against the use of stimulant medications (Chapter 12).

To ensure the comprehensiveness of the rebuttal, I have tried my best to represent the key arguments and beliefs of the consensual biomedical view about ADHD, in a fair manner. Each chapter opens with a careful quotation from a conventional source or known authority in the field, which is then elaborated and given full consideration further in the chapter. I have also made efforts to weave within the refutation, a decent representation of alternative views, which proposed social, cultural, and evolution-oriented explanations for what we call ADHD behaviors. Although the scientific refutation process does not require the proposal of alternative explanations (i.e., the massive empirical evidence contradicting the biomedical view is sufficient to rebut the alleged consensus because it requires us to return to the null hypothesis — see Chapter 1), such views may help us understand how we arrived at such a disturbing situation whereby millions of children are diagnosed with an unreliable psychiatric label and prescribed with ineffective and unsafe medications.

Importantly, **the rebuttal of the consensus brought in this book should not be interpreted as a concrete and personal medical advice**. Any practical decisions should be made cautiously, under proper medical supervision, especially if they involve medications (reducing medications can be a tough, lengthy, and even dangerous process). Bearing this cautionary comment in mind, it is also important to mention another principal ethical rule in medicine, which is the universally accepted norm of *informed consent*. It is our duty, as scientists and practitioners, to provide the public with transparent, wide-scope, and credible information. This is the only way parents could really be given the freedom to choose the best clinical/educational roads for their children, especially considering the fact that these roads are diverged, controversial, and sometimes masked by a thick smoke of conflicts of interest.

Although each chapter may stand on its own, I urge the dear reader to read the book as a whole, in a chronological order, since each step of the refutation, relies, to a certain extent, on its predecessors. Readers should also not miss the final General Discussion section of the book, which illustrates principal insights from the book through a well-documented case study. Moreover, although somewhat outside the scope of the book, this section also outlines key directions for change, that is: short- and long-term actions, that could be taken to improve children's lives, without labeling them with fictitious diagnoses and without prescribing them ineffective and dangerous drugs. Finally, the General Discussion section assembles the numerous validity gaps documented in various parts of the book (Table 4) and offers a holistic picture that refutes the biomedical consensus. In this way, the book that you are about to read may serve as the missing needle that is required to finally pierce the over-blown, and already full-of-holes theoretical balloon known as ADHD.

References

1. Barkley, R.A., *This is how you treat ADHD based off science, Dr Russell Barkley part of 2012 Burnett Lecture*. 2012, keynote lecture at the 2012 Burnett Seminar for Academic Achievement, last retrieved on November 16, 2021, from: https://www.youtube.com/watch?v=_tpB-B8BXk0.
2. Barkley, R.A., *International consensus statement on ADHD*. Journal of the American Academy of Child and Adolescent Psychiatry, 2002. **41**(12): p. 1389.
3. Vos, T., *et al.*, *Global, regional, and national incidence, prevalence, and years lived with disability for 328 diseases and injuries for 195 countries, 1990–2016:*

a systematic analysis for the Global Burden of Disease Study 2016. The Lancet, 2017. **390**(10100): p. 1211–1259.

4. APA, *Diagnostic and Statistical Manual of Mental Disorders (DSM-5®).* 2013: American Psychiatric Association.
5. Faraone, S.V., *The scientific foundation for understanding attention-deficit/hyperactivity disorder as a valid psychiatric disorder.* European Child & Adolescent Psychiatry, 2005. **14**(1): p. 1–10.
6. Kooij, J.J.S., *et al.*, *Updated European Consensus Statement on diagnosis and treatment of adult ADHD.* European Psychiatry, 2019. **56**: p. 14–34.
7. Daley, D., *Attention deficit hyperactivity disorder: a review of the essential facts.* Child Care Health and Development, 2006. **32**(2): p. 193–204.
8. American Academy of Pediatrics, *ADHD: Clinical Practice Guideline for the Diagnosis, Evaluation, and Treatment of Attention-Deficit/Hyperactivity Disorder in Children and Adolescents.* Pediatrics, 2011. **128**(5): p. 1007.
9. Lange, K.W., *et al.*, *The history of attention deficit hyperactivity disorder.* ADHD Attention Deficit and Hyperactivity Disorders, 2010. **2**(4): p. 241–255.
10. Biederman, J. and T. Spencer, *Attention-deficit/hyperactivity disorder (ADHD) as a noradrenergic disorder.* Biological Psychiatry, 1999. **46**(9): p. 1234–1242.
11. Danielson, M.L., *et al.*, *Prevalence of Parent-Reported ADHD Diagnosis and Associated Treatment Among U.S. Children and Adolescents, 2016.* Journal of Clinical Child & Adolescent Psychology, 2018. **47**(2): p. 199–212.
12. Visser, S.N., *et al.*, *Vital signs: national and state-specific patterns of attention deficit/hyperactivity disorder treatment among insured children aged 2–5 years — United States, 2008–2014.* Morbidity and Mortality Weekly Report, 2016. **65**(17): p. 443–450.
13. National Institute of Mental Health, *NIH Consensus Development Conference on Diagnosis and Treatment of Attention Deficit Hyperactivity Disorder: November 16–18, 1998, William H. Natcher Conference Center, National Institutes of Health, Bethesda, Maryland.* 1998: National Institutes of Health, Continuing Medical Education.
14. Bolea-Alamañac, B., *et al.*, *Evidence-based guidelines for the pharmacological management of attention deficit hyperactivity disorder: Update on recommendations*

from the British Association for Psychopharmacology. Journal of Psychopharmacology, 2014. **28**(3): p. 179–203.

15. National Institute for Health and Care Excellence, *Attention deficit hyperactivity disorder: diagnosis and management. NICE Guideline [NG87].* 2018, Last retrieved on August 20, 2021 from: https://www.nice.org.uk/guidance/NG87.
16. Barkley, R.A., *Behavioral inhibition, sustained attention, and executive functions: constructing a unifying theory of ADHD.* Psychological Bulletin, 1997. **121**(1): p. 65.
17. Nigg, J.T., *Is ADHD a disinhibitory disorder?* Psychological bulletin, 2001. **127**(5): p. 571.
18. American Psychiatric Association, *Diagnostic and Statistical Manual of Mental Disorders (DSM-5®).* 2013: American Psychiatric Pub.
19. Barkley, R.A., K.R. Murphy, and M. Fischer, *ADHD in adults: What the science says.* 2010: Guilford press.
20. Engel, G.L., *The need for a new medical model: a challenge for biomedicine.* Science, 1977. **196**(4286): p. 129–136.
21. Lehman, B.J., D.M. David, and J.A. Gruber, *Rethinking the biopsychosocial model of health: Understanding health as a dynamic system.* Social and Personality Psychology Compass, 2017. **11**(8): p. e12328.
22. Schwarz, A., *The selling of attention deficit disorder.* 2013, New York Times, Last retrieved in August, 2021 from: https://www.nytimes.com/2013/12/15/health/the-selling-of-attention-deficit-disorder.html.
23. Carey, W.B. *Is Attention Deficit Hyperactivity Disorder a Valid Disorder?* 1998.
24. Carey, W.B., *Problems in diagnosing attention and activity.* Pediatrics, 1999. **103**(3): p. 664–666.
25. Breggin, P., *The Ritalin fact book: What your doctor won't tell you about ADHD and stimulant drugs.* 2009: Da Capo Lifelong Books.
26. Lambert, N.M. *Stimulant treatment as a risk factor for nicotine use and substance abuse.* 1998.
27. Jensen, P.S., *et al.*, *3-year follow-up of the NIMH MTA study.* Journal of the American Academy of Child & Adolescent Psychiatry, 2007. **46**(8): p. 989–1002.
28. Swanson, J.M., *Debate: Are Stimulant Medications for Attention-Deficit/Hyperactivity Disorder Effective in the Long Term? (Against).* 2019.

29. Lenzer, J., *Review launched after Harvard psychiatrist failed to disclose industry funding.* BMJ, 2008. **336**(7657): p. 1327.
30. Harris, G. and B. Carey, *Researchers fail to reveal full drug pay*, in *New York Times.* 2008, New York Times, Last retrieved on August 26, 2021 from: https://www.nytimes.com/2008/06/08/us/08conflict.html.
31. Timimi, S., *et al., A critique of the international consensus statement on ADHD.* Clinical Child and Family Psychology Review, 2004. **7**(1): p. 59–63; discussion 65–9.
32. Skrabanek, P., *Nonsensus consensus.* The Lancet, 1990. **335**(8703): p. 1446–1447.
33. Timimi, S., *Attention deficit hyperactivity disorder is an example of bad medicine.* Australian & New Zealand Journal of Psychiatry, 2015. **49**(6): p. 575–576.
34. Timimi, S., *The McDonaldization of childhood: Children's mental health in neo-liberal market cultures.* Transcultural Psychiatry, 2010. **47**(5): p. 686–706.
35. Timimi, S. and J. Leo, *Rethinking ADHD: From brain to culture.* 2009: Palgrave.
36. Stolzer, J.M., *Attention deficit hyperactivity disorder: Valid medical condition or culturally constructed myth.* Ethical Human Psychology and Psychiatry, 2009. **11**(1): p. 5–15.
37. Mayes, R., C. Bagwell, and J.L. Erkulwater, *Medicating children: ADHD and pediatric mental health.* 2009: Harvard University Press.
38. Hinshaw, S.P. and R.M. Scheffler, *The ADHD explosion: Myths, medication, money, and today's push for performance.* 2014: Oxford University Press.
39. Smith, M., *Hyperactive Around the World? The History of ADHD in Global Perspective.* Social History of Medicine, 2017. **30**(4): p. 767–787.
40. Corrigan, M.W., *Debunking ADHD: 10 reasons to stop drugging kids for acting like kids.* 2014: Rowman & Littlefield.
41. Maté, G., *Scattered Minds: The Origins and Healing of Attention Deficit Disorder.* 2019: Random House.
42. Harding, B., *The Field Guide to ADHD: What They Don't Want You to Know. Psychiatry — Theory, Applications and Treatments.* Online Submission, 2017.
43. Saul, R., *ADHD Does not Exist: The Truth About Attention Deficit and Hyperactivity Disorder.* 2014: HarperCollins.

44. Spiegel, *What About Tutoring Instead of Pills? Interview with Jerome Kagan.* Spiegel. Last retrieved on June 27, 2021 from: https://www.spiegel.de/international/world/child-psychologist-jerome-kagan-on-overprescibing-drugs-to-children-a-847500.html, 2012.
45. Foreman, D.M., *Attention deficit hyperactivity disorder: legal and ethical aspects.* Archives of Disease in Childhood, 2006. **91**(2): p. 192–194.
46. Parrillo, V.N., *Encyclopedia of social problems.* 2008: Sage Publications.
47. Foreman, D.M. and S. Timimi, *Attention-deficit hyperactivity disorder (ADHD): progress and controversy in diagnosis and treatment.* Irish Journal of Psychological Medicine, 2018. **35**(3): p. 251–257.
48. Mayes, R., C. Bagwell, and J. Erkulwater, *ADHD and the rise in stimulant use among children.* Harvard Review of Psychiatry, 2008. **16**(3): p. 151–166.
49. Merten, E.C., *et al.*, *Overdiagnosis of mental disorders in children and adolescents (in developed countries).* Child and Adolescent Psychiatry and Mental Health, 2017. **11**(1): p. 5.
50. Davidovitch, M., *et al.*, *Diagnosis despite clinical ambiguity: physicians' perspectives on the rise in Autism Spectrum disorder incidence.* BMC Psychiatry, 2021. **21**(1): p. 150.
51. Moncrieff, J. and S. Timimi, *Is ADHD a valid diagnosis in adults? No.* BMJ, 2010. **340**: p. c547.
52. Visser, J. and Z. Jehan, *ADHD: a scientific fact or a factual opinion? A critique of the veracity of Attention Deficit Hyperactivity Disorder.* Emotional and Behavioural Difficulties, 2009. **14**(2): p. 127–140.
53. Armstrong, T., *The Myth of the ADHD Child, Revised Edition: 101 Ways to Improve Your Child's Behavior and Attention Span Without Drugs, Labels, or Coercion.* 2017: Penguin.
54. Maturo, A., *The medicalization of education: ADHD, human enhancement and academic performance.* Italian Journal of Sociology of Education, 2013. **5**(3).
55. Searight, H.R. and A.L. McLaren, *Attention-deficit hyperactivity disorder: The medicalization of misbehavior.* Journal of Clinical Psychology in Medical Settings, 1998. **5**(4): p. 467–495.

Part One

ADHD is Not an Illness:

A step-by-step refutation of the notion
that ADHD is a valid neuropsychiatric disorder

“Real Science Defines ADHD as Real Disorder: Some of the most prestigious scientific-based organizations in the world conclude that ADHD is a real disorder with potentially devastating consequences when not properly identified, diagnosed and treated.”

Children and Adults with ADHD (CHADD). *The Science of ADHD*. Retrieved in November 2021 from CHADD's website [1]

Chapter 1
What makes (any) psychopathology 'real'? The philosophical foundation of the debate

The opening quote of this chapter has been taken from the website of the leading non-profit organization for Children and Adults with ADHD in the US, known as CHADD. According to the organization's description in Facebook, "CHADD is the most trusted source for reliable, science-based information regarding current medical research and ADHD management"; so, when CHADD says that "real science defines ADHD as real disorder", it contributes to the dismissal of the vibrant debate over the validity of the diagnosis presented in the Introduction. Moreover, the usage of the terms "real science" and "real disorder" might create an inaccurate impression among non-scientists, as if Attention Deficit Hyperactivity Disorder (ADHD) is a *physiological* disorder — a unique neurodevelopmental construct that is distinguished from the rest of the *mental* disorders. The biomedical conceptualization of ADHD as a chronic "brain disorder" or as "the diabetes of psychiatry" (Introduction) may lead people to believe that ADHD can be diagnosed through objective biological measures that prove, without a doubt, that the person *has* a tangible brain deficit. However, the truth is that ADHD does not have any physiological advantage over other mental health disorders (Chapter 6).

Complexity and subjectivity in psychopathology

Like all other psychopathologies, the clinical diagnosis of ADHD relies mainly on behavioral observations and subjective questionnaires. Indeed, some clinicians use more objective (yet, non-physiological) computer-based Continuous Performance Tests (CPTs), but these neuropsychological tests are considered even less valid than the more traditional self-report scales [2]. A thorough discussion of the validity of these tests, as well as the validity of the principal claims regarding the neurobiological underpinnings of ADHD is provided in Chapter 6, but for the purpose of the current opening chapter, let me cite only the general diagnostic rule of the *Diagnostic and Statistical Manual of Mental Disorders* (*DSM*) according to which: "in the absence of clear biological markers... it has not been possible to completely separate normal and pathological symptom expressions contained in diagnostic criteria" [3, p. 21].

In contrast to popular biological deterministic views, the promising biological revolution in psychiatry of the previous century has not lived up to its expectations [4]. At this time, as articulated in a recent editorial article in *JAMA Psychiatry* (the leading psychiatric journal of the American Medical Association), it seems that "we are standing at a precipice: our explanatory disease models are woefully insufficient, and our predictive approaches have not yielded robust individual-level predictions that can be used by clinicians" [5]. Critics of the simplistic biological views are continuously reminding us that (as of today) human behaviors and experiences cannot be reduced to a small number of biological elements [6]. Not only does this biological reductionism have negligible predictive value for clinical diagnosis, it could lead to "*diagnostic literalism*" — a problematic perception of abstract and tentative human-drafted labels as concrete and real medical entities [7, 8]. Psychiatric conditions are much better understood from a more complex ecological point of view, as products of multifaceted interactions between a wide range of biological, psychological, interpersonal, and environmental factors [9, 10]. Simplistic biomedically-inspired assertions, such as: "Simba behaves this way because he *has* ADHD," therefore have very little clinical value or real scientific truth.

Furthermore, even if one day, ADHD-like behaviors will be proven to originate from clear biological components, these components have very little relevance to real-life clinical diagnoses. The fundamental monistic approach (see Chapter 6) that is shared by most scientists is that all human experiences, even the most amorphic ones, have some physiological manifestation in the brain. High intellectual abilities, for example, might be expressed in physical brain activity somehow, but, of course, we will not argue that brain differences between geniuses and non-geniuses are indicative of a pathology. Similarly, brain differences between males and females do not necessarily mean that one of the genders has impaired brains. Thus, to answer the question "whether ADHD is real", we should take a theoretical step backwards and understand the basic philosophical assumptions that stand behind the conceptualization of mental disorders. In other words, we need to ask: What makes various human behaviors a valid psychiatric disorder?

The "Four Ds" criteria of psychiatric diagnosis

Usually, the starting point of the deliberation, whether certain behaviors constitute a mental disorder (i.e., psychopathology), is a series of indications that the explored behaviors appear together, in a relatively holistic form (i.e., convergent validity) and that this holistic form is distinct from other clusters of behaviors (i.e., discriminant validity). The convergence of several behaviors (e.g., "often makes careless mistakes", "often has difficulty organizing tasks") into a unified and statistically distinct cluster of behaviors (e.g., inattentiveness) may attest that this cluster originates from a genuine psychiatric condition, thus lending support to the *construct validity* of the proposed theory regarding the disorder (see Box 1 for a brief description of the various types of reliability and validity in psychological assessment and empirical research). As will be seen in Chapter 5, this basic requirement is not really met in ADHD; however, even if it is and distinctive clusters of inattentive/hyperactive behaviors do exist, we still need to determine whether these behaviors are abnormal, yet alone, pathological.

Throughout history, humans have tried to understand and classify abnormal behaviors [11]. From a philosophy of science point of view, the premise of this investigation — the *null hypothesis (H0)* as it is commonly referred as — is the assumption that **human beings are normal until proven otherwise**, regardless of whether they are, for example, homosexual, energetic, or introverted. In order to reject the null hypothesis and argue for an *alternative hypothesis (H1)*, in which a cluster of behaviors constitute a psychiatric disorder, theorists must first prove that these traits are exceptionally deviant from normal human behaviors, meaning that they are at the extreme end of the human behavior spectrum (also see Chapter 2). In fact, this is only the first criterion that must be met before subsequent criteria are considered.

A conventional and easy to remember typology that helps us determine whether given behaviors form a mental disorder is the *"Four Ds" criteria of psychiatric diagnosis*, consisting of Deviance, Dysfunction, Danger, and Distress [12]. As mentioned above, the first *criterion of Deviance* is considered a prerequisite condition for labeling a person with a psychiatric condition. Behaviors, cognitions, and emotions can only be abnormal if they are **not** normal, that is, that they deviate from the normal distribution. Moreover, even if a certain behavior is deviant from the perspective of one cultural group (e.g., talking to invisible entities), it may not be deviant in another cultural group. Believe it or not, a person who invites angels to bless his family on a Friday night may be considered perfectly normal within his community and we do not need to call an ambulance. In other words, it is not enough that we (society, clinicians) declare that a certain behavior is deviant; we need to make sure that the behavior is abnormal within the close context of the person's life and remember that different groups have different values and norms. Fascinatingly, the *DSM* goes even a step further and warns that "socially deviant behavior (e.g., political, religious, or sexual) and conflicts that are primarily between the individual and society are **not** mental disorders unless **the deviance or conflict results from a dysfunction in the individual**" [3, p. 20; bold added by Y.O.].

Then, after we have established the exceptionality of the behaviors, we still need to prove the existence of all or most of the remaining three Ds. Humans naturally differ from one another; some are extremely energetic, some are exceptionally social, and some even love broccoli. This *neurodiversity* may actually be the basis of what we call a talent [13, 14]. Genius, for example, by definition, meets the criterion of statistical deviance, yet it is not indicative of psychopathology (for more information, see Chapter 2). To define a human behavior as a mental disorder, we must prove that the given behavioral pattern significantly impairs the person's ability to lead a normative life. This is most often assessed by examining the severity of the three additional criteria: Dysfunction, Distress, and Danger.

The *criterion of Dysfunction* is usually manifested in significant impairments that occur in simple, daily functioning, such as dressing, eating, or showering. Maladaptive behaviors that cause these dysfunctions and prevent a person from living a healthy life without being dependent on others for a constant help may indeed deserve a psychiatric label (assuming that they are not a product of a known physical condition). But even this strong criterion may not suffice. Consider, for example, a person who chooses to go on a hunger strike in protest, or even a person who chooses not to go to work. Can these 'dysfunctions', by themselves, be used as a conclusive sign that the person suffers from a mental disorder?

A third, and more subjective criterion, is therefore needed, the *criterion of Distress*. In most mental disorders, we assume that the persons *suffer* from their condition; that the deviant behaviors or cognitions they exhibit, cause them (subjective) emotional or physical pain. This criterion may be tricky because some people may embrace or hold positive attitudes towards their deviant behaviors even if they are clearly maladaptive for them, such as in some cases of Anorexia Nervosa. In this criterion, we therefore need to explore the person's feelings deeply and try to understand what he/she thinks about his/her behaviors. Are the behaviors more *egosyntonic*, that is, in harmony with the person's expectations and lifegoals, or more *egodystonic*, that is, posing mainly agony, conflict, and stress?

Finally, the last *criterion of Danger*, although less prevalent in psychiatric diagnosis, should also be investigated. The anorexic girl may sanctify her non-eating practices, but these practices can put her life in danger or trigger further health risks. She may therefore be eligible for a psychiatric diagnosis even if she insists that she does not feel any emotional distress. It is noted that the danger criterion should be considered both for the person with the dangerous behaviors and for people in her/his surroundings. Individuals who experience severely depressive feelings might meet the criterion of danger because they can harm themselves. Individuals with recurrent delusional paranoias might meet the criterion of danger because their delusions might lead them to hurt people in their surroundings (unfortunately, these people can be their closest caring friends or family). Highly dangerous behaviors can therefore be indicative of a pathology, but once again, they cannot be considered as a sufficient condition for determining that a person suffers from a mental disorder. Otherwise, all murderers or extreme sport lovers would be eligible for a psychiatric diagnosis.

The main idea behind this Four Ds conceptualization is that we should be careful not to determine that a person has a disorder, based on a narrow prism of plain human difficulties or conflicts. Of course, not all these criteria must be fully met in any given disorder. There is often a trade-off between the various criteria. For example, a phenomenon that causes severe impairment in functioning, such as Intellectual Disability, does not necessarily meet the danger criterion. Alternatively, a phenomenon that puts the person in imminent risk of suicide does not necessarily cause daily dysfunction. Essentially, in order to claim that certain behaviors constitute a psychiatric disorder, it is necessary to verify that the statistically deviant set of behaviors produces a serious and significant impairment to the person's ability to lead a normative life. Correspondingly, the *DSM* definition of a mental disorder is "a syndrome characterized by clinically significant disturbance in an individual's cognition, emotion regulation, or behavior" [3, p. 20]. Mental disorders, according to the manual "are usually associated with significant distress or disability in social, occupational, or other important activities". However, even if a significant distress or disability exists, the manual defines a key constraint. "An expectable or culturally approved response to a common stressor… is **not** a mental disorder" (p. 20).

Taken together, in order to determine that attention difficulties and/or hyperactivity behaviors constitute a mental disorder, we are required to consider the existence and severity of the above Four Ds criteria and ensure that the individual's difficulties are "a dysfunction in the individual" and are not an "expectable response to a common stressor". The following chapters explore the relevance of these fundamental diagnostic criteria to the neuropsychiatric condition we call ADHD. Only through a detailed exploration of these criteria could we assess the validity of the opening assertion of this chapter according to which: "Real Science Defines ADHD as Real Disorder."

Box 1 — Reliability and validity in scientific research

The term *reliability* usually refers to our ability to measure variables accurately and consistently with as few errors as possible. There are various types of reliability, including: *stability over time*, *inter-rater reliability*, and *internal consistency*. Reliability is a prerequisite condition for further validity (see below) of concepts (e.g., research variables) and for any research findings and conclusions that are based on empirical assessment. That is, when there is a problem of reliability in the measurement phase of the research, then there ought to be a problem with the validity of the findings and the conclusions drawn from that research [15].

The term *validity* usually refers to the extent to which the variable itself (e.g., ADHD), the means of assessing its existence and severity (i.e., observations and measurement tools), and the findings and conclusions drawn from the research targeting this variable, are all based on solid scientific foundations, which correspond with reality [16]. Validity is a central concept both in psychological assessment and in empirical research.

In psychological assessment, the term validity refers to the extent to which an observational tool (e.g., Conner's rating scale for assessing ADHD) accurately measures the theoretical variable it is intended to measure (e.g., ADHD). There are several types of measurement validity, including *predictive validity*, *content validity*, and *construct validity*. Note that, although the last term (construct validity) usually refers to issues in psychological testing, this book uses this term in its broader meaning to also describe theoretical issues that are not related directly to psychological assessment (e.g., when the theory dictates something, and the empirical evidence suggests the opposite). Generally speaking, the term construct validity refers to the degree to which there is a fit between the observed variable and the theoretical construct of that variable [17]. Specifically, construct validity consists of two types of validity known as *discriminant validity* and *convergent validity* — the degree to which the measurement items or the observed behaviors form a unified cluster (i.e., convergent validity) that is clearly distinct from other clusters (i.e., discriminant validity).

In empirical research, the term *internal validity* refers to the extent to which conclusions can be drawn about relationships (particularly causal relationships) between the various variables of the research, based on the measurement tools, the research sample, the experimental design, and the applied quantitative or qualitative analyses [16]. In order to reach valid (causal) conclusions and avoid spurious or false findings, the gold standard in psychological and medical research is a longitudinal Randomized Control Trial (RCT), which is conducted in an objective ("blind") manner, with as few conflicts of interest as possible. Poor quality research (e.g., non-controlled cross-sectional studies) and high risk of bias impair our ability to derive valid conclusions. Like the previous validity type, this book refers to internal validity in its broader meaning, to also evaluate the strength of a given argument within the theory (e.g., poor internal validity is attributed to arguments that are not empirically or logically supported).

The term *ecological validity* refers to the extent to which research results are relevant to real-life situations, outside of the research framework. This type of validity is central for the generalizability of research findings to other populations, settings, situations, and times [18].

Note that Table 4 at the General Discussion section outlines the various reliability and validity gaps that exist in the current conceptualization of ADHD and its associated pharmacological treatments.

References

1. CHADD, *The Science of ADHD*. Retreived in November 2021, CHADD: Children and Adults with ADHD, 4221 Forbes Blvd, Suite 270, Lanham, MD, 20706. Last retrieved on November 16, 2021 from: https://chadd.org/about-adhd/the-science-of-adhd/.
2. Barkley, R.A., *Neuropsychological testing is not useful in the diagnosis of ADHD: Stop it (or prove it)!* The ADHD Report, 2019. **27**(2): p. 1–8.
3. APA, *Diagnostic and Statistical Manual of Mental Disorders (DSM-5®)*. 2013: American Psychiatric Association.
4. Harrington, A., *Mind fixers: Psychiatry's troubled search for the biology of mental illness*. 2019: WW Norton & Company.
5. Paulus, M.P. and W.K. Thompson, *The Challenges and Opportunities of Small Effects: The New Normal in Academic Psychiatry.* JAMA Psychiatry, 2019. **76**(4): p. 353–354.
6. Rosenberg, C.E., *Contested boundaries: psychiatry, disease, and diagnosis.* Perspectives in biology and Medicine, 2006. **49**(3): p. 407–424.
7. Kendler, K.S., *DSM disorders and their criteria: how should they inter-relate?* Psychological Medicine, 2017. **47**(12): p. 2054–2060.
8. Fried, E.I., *Studying mental disorders as systems, not syndromes.* PsyArXiv, 2021.
9. Lehman, B.J., D.M. David, and J.A. Gruber, *Rethinking the biopsychosocial model of health: Understanding health as a dynamic system.* Social and Personality Psychology Compass, 2017. **11**(8): p. e12328.
10. Engel, G.L., *The need for a new medical model: a challenge for biomedicine.* Science, 1977. **196**(4286): p. 129–136.
11. Blashfield, R.K., *et al.*, *The cycle of classification: DSM-I through DSM-5.* Annual Review of Clinical Psychology, 2014. **10**: p. 25–51.
12. Davis, T.O., *Conceptualizing Psychiatric Disorders Using 'Four D's' of Diagnoses.* The Internet Journal of Psychiatry, 2009. **1**(1): p. 1.
13. Armstrong, T., *The Power of Neurodiversity: Unleashing the Advantages of Your Differently Wired Brain (published in hardcover as Neurodiversity).* 2011: Da Capo Lifelong Books.

14. McGee, M., *Neurodiversity.* Contexts, 2012. **11**(3): p. 12–13.
15. Holt, N.J., *et al., Psychology: The science of mind and behaviour.* 2012: McGraw-Hill Education.
16. Brewer, M.B. and W.D. Crano, *Research design and issues of validity.* Handbook of research methods in social and personality psychology, 2000: p. 3–16.
17. Cronbach, L.J. and P.E. Meehl, *Construct validity in psychological tests.* Psychological Bulletin, 1955. **52**(4): p. 281.
18. Mitchell, M.L. and J.M. Jolley, *Research design explained.* 2012: Cengage Learning.

“

- “ADHD occurs in about 5% of children” (Mohammadi et al., 2021) [1].
- “Prevalence of ADHD ranges between 5.29% and 7.1%” (Joshi & Angolkar, 2021) [2].
- “Prevalence of ADHD is 6.5% in childhood” (Sandstrom et al., 2021) [3].
- “Approximately 9.4% of children aged 2 to 17 have been diagnosed with ADHD” (Wong & Landes, 2021) [4].

Chapter 2
Does ADHD meet the criterion of Deviance?

We begin our inquiry of the "Four Ds" criteria of psychiatric diagnosis (Chapter 1), with the first and prerequisite criterion of Deviance. Like all other psychiatric disorders, we expect that cases of Attention Deficit Hyperactivity Disorder (ADHD) will be relatively uncommon, otherwise the behaviors associated with the disorder could not have been categorized as abnormal. In fact, the very use of the term '*Hyperactivity*' indicates that there are normative levels of activity and 'hyper' (i.e., above normal) levels of activity. In other words, by definition, ADHD is conceptualized as a deviant phenomenon. The mission of the current chapter should therefore be relatively simple (especially considering the consensual, biomedical perception of ADHD) — to investigate two straightforward questions: What is the prevalence of ADHD-related behaviors in the general population and to what extent do these behaviors deviate from normal human behaviors? Nevertheless, as illustrated in the opening quotes of this chapter, the answers to these questions may not be so simple. Although all four quotations were taken from new articles published in the same year (2021), and although all four served as opening statements that supposedly reflect a well-established truth about the prevalence of ADHD, they still present significantly different prevalence estimates (e.g., 5% vs. 9.4%). Moreover, even if we manage to settle these discrepancies and scrutinize the exact rates of ADHD, how do we decide whether these rates are deviant? After all, human beings differ from one another on multiple traits, and to my knowledge, there is no formal quantitative cutoff point at which all agree that a given trait or behavior deviates from the standard norm.

The deviance criterion in neurodevelopmental disorders

Without a formal cutoff point for deviant behaviors, perhaps we could compare the debated disorder of ADHD to other mental disorders of childhood, preferably to disorders with similar etiological assumptions, that is: disorders that are conceptualized as biological-originated, lifelong deficits. A classic example for a statistically based deviance can be found in Intellectual Disability (Intellectual Developmental Disorder) — a neighboring disorder that shares the same *Diagnostic and Statistical Manual of Mental Disorders* (*DSM*)-clustering with ADHD (i.e., the cluster of neurodevelopmental disorders). The first criterion of Intellectual Disability — the wide-ranging deficit in intellectual functions — is usually measured by validated Intelligence Quotient (IQ) tests [5]. Based on the assumption that IQ levels are normally distributed in the general population, it is agreed that the five percent that comprises the two extreme ends of the distribution represents a population that significantly deviates from the norm (see Figure 1 for a schematic illustration). In other words, approximately 95% of the population have IQ levels within two Standard Deviations (SD) from the average level, 2.5% have IQ levels that are extremely high, and 2.5% have IQ levels that are extremely low and can therefore be indicative of a deficit in intellectual functioning.

At a first glance, a standard deviation score of 2 points, which comprises only 2.5% of the population may serve as a good rule of thumb for determining that a given behavior, or a trait (whether positive or negative), meets the prerequisite criterion of deviance. Correspondingly, the seminal Milwaukee Longitudinal Study of Hyperactive (ADHD) Children conducted by Prof.

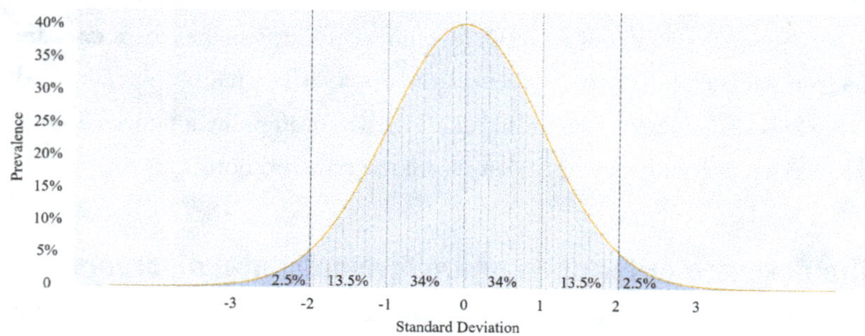

Figure 1. A schematic illustration of a normal distribution

Barkley himself (see the Introduction), used a cut-off point of two standard deviations above the mean for severity of symptoms to allocate children to the experimental group of the study [6]. However, even this rule is not always sufficient, as can be learnt from the case of Intellectual Disability. As mentioned in Chapter 1, the definition of a psychiatric disorder depends not only on how rare a phenomenon is, but also on the extent to which the deviant behaviors or traits (i.e., the low IQ levels) impair the person's ability to lead a normal life. This straightforward convention may explain why the actual prevalence of Intellectual Disability is estimated to be around 1%, rather than 2.5%, and why the prevalence of Severe Intellectual Disability is only about 6 per 1000 [5, p. 38].

It is noted that in the context of the *DSM* neurodevelopmental cluster of disorders, even 1% can be seen as a suspiciously large number. The prevalence of Autism Spectrum Disorder, another neighboring disorder that shares the cluster with ADHD, has only approached the troubling rates of 1% in the current edition of the psychiatric manual (*DSM*-5). The reasons for this increase are still being investigated [7], but even the *DSM* seems to recognize the possibility that the prevalence of 1% may not reflect the true rates of the disorder. According to the *DSM*, two artifacts might have inflated the rates of the diagnosis: an artificial expansion of the previous diagnostic criteria, which now includes "subthreshold cases," and differences in the measuring tools that were used in the various studies on Autism Spectrum Disorder [5, p. 55]. Correspondingly, a large percent of expert clinicians believe that Autism Spectrum Disorder is over-diagnosed [8].

The consensual prevalence of 5% in ADHD

Bearing the aforementioned rates in mind, we can now start to consider whether the reported rates of ADHD meet the first criterion of *abnormal* behavior (i.e., deviance). We shall start this consideration with the official rates of the disorder, as reported in the *DSM*. According to this authoritative medical source: "ADHD occurs in most cultures in about 5% of children and about 2.5% of adults"

[5, p. 61]. These estimates correspond (to a certain extent) with a highly cited systematic review of 102 epidemiological studies published between 1978 and 2005, which documented a worldwide-pooled prevalence of 5.29% [9]. Somewhat similar figures were reported in the more recent consensus statement regarding adult ADHD: “In childhood, ADHD is among **the most common psychiatric disorders** with a prevalence rate of 3–5%... the prevalence of ADHD in adults across twenty countries was recently estimated at 2.8%, with a range between 1.4–3.6%” [10, p. 20; bold added by Y.O.].

Although these numbers represent a relatively conservative prevalence estimate, compared with other, well-documented reports (see below), they are still very disturbing in my view. If these numbers are true, then at least tens of millions of children worldwide are suffering from this alleged lifelong neurodevelopmental impairment [11, 12]. In other words, even before attempting to explain the higher rates that are reported in updated national surveys, it can be said that ADHD, a highly “common psychiatric disorder” of childhood, is *not* really a deviant phenomenon, especially considering the proposed rule of thumb (i.e., 2 standard deviations units) mentioned earlier, and the reported rates of other chronic, neurodevelopmental conditions, which do not exceed 1%.

The dramatic increase in ADHD rates

Truth be told, the prevalence estimate of the *DSM* was not always so high. When the disorder was first introduced in 1980, in the third edition of the diagnostic manual (*DSM*-III), as “Attention Deficit” (rather than the non-attention focused labels used beforehand), the prevalence estimate of the disorder was 3%, and even back then, the disorder was considered “common” [13, p. 42]. Nowadays of course, there is accumulating evidence that ADHD has become extremely common. There appears to be a consistent annual increase in the number of children and adolescents diagnosed with ADHD. In the US for example, between the years 2003 and 2011, the prevalence of the diagnosis has soared by 42% [14]. Indeed, different studies report different rates, but according to the relatively reliable National Survey of Children's Health (NSCH), conducted by the US Centers for Disease Control and Prevention (CDC) in 2016, a total of 9.6% of all children (6–11 years) and 13.6% of all adolescents (12–17 years), had ever received a medical diagnosis of ADHD [15]. Worryingly, at age 12, the prevalence estimate has been documented to exceed the **20% point** among boys — a troubling estimate that replicates the previous national survey findings, according to which ADHD rates exceeded 20% among boys aged 11-14 years [14]. These exceptional figures are particularly troubling in light of the consensual notions that the foundation of ADHD is neurological, rather than sociological [16], and that ADHD occurs "in most cultures" at about the same rate [5, p. 61].

It is important to acknowledge that the troubling rates of ADHD are not an 'American problem' only. Multiple studies from places around the world have documented prevalence rates that significantly exceed the 3-5% estimates of the various editions of the *DSM*. High estimates of ADHD range from: 12.6% in Egypt [17], 17.1% in Colombia [18], 17.3% in Iran [19], 17.8% in Germany [20], 18% in Brazil [21], and 19.8% in Ukraine [22]. Of note is a very recent large Israeli study that did not address the epidemiology of ADHD directly, but accidently revealed that between 18.85% to 28.14% of children and young adults (5–20 years) were clinically diagnosed with ADHD [23]. What makes these findings from Israel powerful is the fact that they rely on thousands of formal medical records, that are real clinical diagnoses of ADHD, rather than on subjective self-report screening tools (for more information about this study, see Chapter 12).

I am not arguing that the aforementioned studies from various parts of the world represent the average global prevalence of ADHD. The heterogeneity of the available epidemiological research is huge [9, 12] and different studies report substantially different rates of ADHD (a reliability problem on its own, which is discussed later in this chapter). However, I do believe that these numbers require more scientific attention, since even proponents of the disorder are starting to acknowledge these high rates, thus admitting that ADHD tends to be over-diagnosed unjustifiably [8].

To further examine the reliability of the skyrocketing figures of ADHD, I have conducted three consecutive empirical studies myself: Study 1 and Study 2 addressed young adults aged 18–30, while Study 3 focused on mothers of school-aged children during the COVID-19 pandemic [24]. The general goal of these studies was to investigate whether the biomedical perception of ADHD is indeed grounded and manifested in our daily reality (and I will return to the findings of these studies in various parts of this book) and I have started this investigation with a simple research question: What is the actual prevalence of ADHD today, in Israel?

To answer this seemingly simple question however, we should first overcome a known problem in the epidemiology of a lifetime disorder. Aside from methodological differences (e.g., different assessment tools), one of the reasons for the high heterogeneity in the epidemiological literature on ADHD may be the choice of some researchers to investigate the prevalence of the diagnosis at the present moment, among a given cohort of participants. However, when researchers examine a cohort of elementary school children, for example, they might miss the children who will be diagnosed later in their life, during high school or college. Consider for example, a recent longitudinal study that was published in *JAMA*, the leading Journal of the American Medical Association [25]. In this study, the authors excluded 6.9% of their original sample of 2,843 adolescents, because these participants were screened positive for ADHD at baseline and the authors wished to explore the effects of digital media use on non-ADHD adolescents. They then discovered, six months later, that another 6.9% of the remaining non-ADHD sample experienced ADHD symptoms (of which, by the way, a large percentage could not be explained through the prism of digital media use).

The implied hypothesis of the above study, according to which environmental factors, such as digital media use can lead to ADHD, is by its own, somewhat contradicting to the biogenetic conceptualization of the disorder as an innate brain deficit (also, are we heading towards a dystopic future whereby most children will be infected with ADHD because of the ubiquitous spread of digital media technologies?). But let's put this construct validity problem aside for the moment and return to the biomedical consensus.

If ADHD is indeed an innate lifelong neurogenetic deficit that cannot be diagnosed without evident symptoms at a very young age (Introduction), then individuals who received the diagnosis later in life (e.g., during college) must have had an undetected version of the disorder as children. Studies that rely on self-report diagnoses at the present moment are therefore bound to yield underestimated rates of ADHD. In other words, the underlying assumption of the scientific consensus is that the prevalence of the diagnosis is accumulative: The percent of individuals who are diagnosed during adolescence or adulthood in a given cohort should be added to the existing percent of individuals who were diagnosed as children.

Since I did not have the resources to conduct a longitudinal study (it is not easy to secure funding for 'heretical' research which does not align with the consensus), I chose to target this problem through a retrospective research on young adults, rather than a prospective study on children [24]. In Study 1 and Study 2, I have asked adult participants to indicate whether they had ever received a formal medical diagnosis of ADHD in the past (in Study 2, they were also asked to complete a formal ADHD scale). This data collection strategy proved to be justified, as more than half of all the diagnosed participants in these studies received their first ADHD diagnosis during, or after, their adolescence. The average age of first diagnosis was about 13.5 in both studies and over 10% received their first diagnosis only after they reached adulthood, at the age of 18 years or older. To somehow address this issue in Study 3, which focused on children, mothers of school-aged children were given an option to indicate whether they believe that one or more of their children have ADHD, even though none of them were formally diagnosed. To ensure the validity of all three studies, a strict data quality assurance protocol was applied [26] and only attentive participants who passed subtle attention checks and rigid quality measures were included in the analyses.

At the beginning, when I started receiving the data from Study 1, which was collected for me by a neutral and well-acknowledged national survey service without any awareness of the purpose of the study, I couldn't believe my own dataset. In this short study, a national representative sample of Jewish participants were only asked to indicate if they had ever received one or more of the following medical diagnoses: Attention Deficit Hyperactivity Disorder (ADHD), Schizophrenia, Autism Spectrum Disorder, Depressive Disorder, and Social Anxiety (multiple answers were allowed). Participants who reported of ADHD diagnosis were subsequently asked to indicate how old they were when they first received the diagnosis. The findings were astonishing: A total of **23.1%** of the representative sample reported that they received a diagnosis of ADHD. Remarkably, the diagnosis of ADHD was far more prevalent than the four other potential diagnoses of: Schizophrenia (0.4%), Autism Spectrum Disorder (0.4%), Depressive Disorder (6.0%), and Social Anxiety (5.2%). While the observed rates of the four other diagnoses were lower or equivalent to the *DSM*-5 estimates (0.3-0.7%, 1%, 7%, 7%, for Schizophrenia, Autism Spectrum Disorder, Depressive Disorder, and Social Anxiety, respectively), the observed rates of ADHD disproportionally exceeded the *DSM* estimates. A Chi-Square test, whereby the expected value for ADHD has been set to 0.05, as suggested by the *DSM*, showed that this difference between the observed prevalence and the *DSM* estimate is significant and extremely large (X^2 = 346.522, $p < 0.001$, *Cohen's d* = 2.98).

Similar large gaps were found in the subsequent two studies as well. Study 2 focused on undergraduate students from two large Israeli colleges who were recruited in a snowball sampling process (in contrast to the randomized representative sampling of Study 1). Aside from answering the same question from Study 1 regarding the formal diagnosis of ADHD, participants in this study were also asked to complete several more questionnaires, including a short version of the World Health Organization (WHO) Adult ADHD Self-Report Scale (ASRS) [27] and a customized questionnaire that addressed their subjective perceptions of the disorder and their use of ADHD medications (for more information about these questionnaires, see Chapters 3 and 5). Here, the findings regarding the prevalence of ADHD were even more troubling. Over 30% of the participating students reported they received a diagnosis of ADHD in the past. Indeed, the rates in this study may be inflated compared with the representative sample of Study 1 due to the snowball sampling method and the mostly non-religious population of the sample (for the contributing factor of religious affiliation, see further in this chapter). However, they too indicate that the 5% estimate of the *DSM* does not characterize "most cultures" today. Study 3, which focused on children, corroborated these high rates, and suggested that almost half of all households include at least one child with either diagnosed ADHD (29.4%) or with ADHD-like behaviors (19.3%) that lead mothers to suspect they have (yet-to-be diagnosed) ADHD.

Obviously, my local Israeli studies are not without limitations. Although data quality assurance methods were applied, participants' responses may not provide the most accurate reflection of the current status of the diagnosis in Israel, especially in the non-representative sample of Study 2. Moreover, it is possible that Israel is leading the world (together with some other Western-oriented countries) in diagnosis and treatment rates of ADHD [28], thus challenging our ability to generalize the findings to other countries. Nevertheless, even if my prevalence estimates are unique to Israel or randomly inflated, they raise a complex public health question: How is it possible that the prevalence of a neurogenetic condition that "occurs in most cultures in about 5% of children", increased in some places to such high rates? Are some populations at a greater risk for this biogenetic disorder?

The ever-changing rates of ADHD

To answer the last question, we first need to explore the validity of the notion that ADHD occurs in most cultures in about the same rate. Apparently, the rates of ADHD differ, both between, and within countries. Data from the US, for examples, indicated large diagnostic gaps between states, which ranged from 5.6% in Nevada to 15.6% in North Carolina [29]. Moreover, findings from the 2011 National Survey of Children's Health showed that the rates of ADHD are **dependent on almost every examined sociodemographic variable** [14] including: *Gender* (15.1% for boys vs. 6.7% for girls); *Age* (14.3% for 11–14 years vs. 7.7% for 4–10 years); *Race and Ethnicity* (e.g., 12.2% for White vs. 6.0% for Hispanic/Latino); and *Geographic region* (e.g.,

12.6% in the South vs. 8.1% in the West). High rates of ADHD were also evidenced among children from *English-speaking households*, children with *high school graduated parents*, and children from *low income families* [14]. In other words, contrary to the biomedical paradigm, cultural, sociological, and even political factors may play a significant role in the diagnosis of ADHD [30-32]. The first two central sociodemographic factors of age and gender, which were repeatedly shown to impact the prevalence of ADHD, are discussed further in this book in the contexts of the dysfunction criterion (Chapter 3) and the danger criterion (Chapter 4). The third central factor of culture is discussed below.

The underestimated role of cultural affiliation

Apparently, minority groups that do not share the dominant values and norms of the majority tend to have lower rates of ADHD [14, 15]. Both of the aforementioned CDC national surveys found that Hispanic/Latino populations had lower rates of ADHD compared to white populations. Correspondingly, a new study found that the prevalence of the diagnosis is significantly lower among Hispanic and Asian children, compared with Non-Hispanic White children [4]. It is possible then, that sociological perceptions about children's 'right' behaviors are involved in the diagnosis of this alleged brain deficit. In my own studies (Study 1 and Study 2), I have evidenced a consistent and significant pattern according to which, the less conservative the person is, the more likely that she/he will be diagnosed with ADHD [24]. In Israel, the Jewish population can be classified to four relatively distinct levels of religiosity: Secular (not-religious individuals), Traditional (not-religious individuals who maintain key religious customs), Orthodox (observant Jews), and Ultra-orthodox (devout observant Jews that are called 'Haredim'). These groups showed a consistent linear trend in ADHD rates: Whereas only 6.7% of the ultra-orthodox sector received a diagnosis of ADHD in the representative sample of Study 1, 16.4% were diagnosed in the orthodox sector, 25.7% in the traditional sector, and 26.0% in the secular sector ($\beta = .48, p = .001$).

Without objective measures and criteria for ADHD (e.g., "often runs about or climbs"), different religious/traditional communities can easily determine their own (implicit) cutoff points for the diagnosis (i.e., what level of unwanted behaviors should be considered as pathological and be referred to further medical examination). Some communities may be more tolerant to ADHD-like behaviors and accept them as normal children's conduct, while others may be less tolerant and prefer to label them as a medical condition. In the same vein, some communities may encourage school/college students to achieve a medical diagnosis of ADHD to be eligible for treatments that are thought to improve the students' performance, while others may encourage students to cope with life challenges without medical interventions. Evangelical Christians for example, are more suspicious towards the medical diagnosis and treatment of ADHD compared with the general population [33]. This specific group seems to avoid pharmacological interventions that, in their view, disguise the real therapeutic work that should be done within the family unit. Either way, the resultant medical diagnosis is not given to the individual based on an accurate estimation of an objective neurogenetic deficit and "the deviance or [the] conflict" do not seem to "result from a dysfunction in the individual", as required by the *DSM* (Chapter 1). On the contrary, in many cases, ADHD-related behaviors seem to reflect "conflicts that are primarily between the individual and [the] society", as will be illustrated further in this chapter, as well as in Chapters 3 and 5.

The oppression of the poor

A second, and in my opinion, very disturbing sociological phenomenon that should be voiced over and over again is the fact that some minorities and underprivileged children are being medically labeled more than others. Low-income families and black populations, for example, are consistently documented to have relatively high rates of ADHD [14, 15]. Are we indeed willing to claim that these groups are more prone to suffer from a neurodevelopmental condition? Take for example, the studies that documented lower Intelligence Quotient (IQ) levels among certain races and ethnicities and among low income families [e.g., 34]. Would scientists dare to claim that these studies provide evidence for white/rich intelligence supremacy? Similarly, in many places, women earn less than men [e.g., 35]. Does this mean that their work is less productive? How come we all agree that in these cases, the origin of the differences is social and not biological, but we refuse to do so (i.e., acknowledge the role of sociology) in the case of ADHD?

Of course, many white and rich individuals also receive the diagnosis of ADHD, as can be vividly seen in various prestigious colleges [24], but it seems that their underlying reason for getting the diagnosis is different. Whereas some individuals and parents request the diagnosis willingly (perhaps to enjoy some educational benefits of the label or to achieve access to prescribed medications), others — less privileged individuals (mainly children) — may be almost forced to get the diagnosis by their surroundings. It is possible that some schools and medical personnel have less tolerance towards disruptive behaviors of children of color or of low-income families (see also my Personal Prologue). Instead of offering compassion to these children, they send them a deterministic message, whether explicitly or implicitly, that something is wrong with their brains, and that they ought to take medications, otherwise they could not fit in. Unfortunately, the parents (and sometimes the single parent mother) do not always have the power to resist this deterministic message, so they unwillingly surrender to the pressure exerted on them.

The epidemiology of ADHD contradicts the biomedical paradigm

Astonishingly, when 'believers' of the disorder are confronted with such claims regarding the unexplainable rise in ADHD rates and the instability of the diagnosis, some of them argue that environmental factors are indeed involved in the etiology of ADHD, thus challenging its purely biogenetic nature, and essentially requiring us to revisit our entire understanding of the disorder (see the aforementioned study that linked ADHD rates with digital media use). Other 'believers' prefer to dismiss the evidence regarding the rise in ADHD rates and insist that, not only is the diagnosis stable over time and across most cultures, it is also in fact, **underdiagnosed** in the real world [10, 36, 37].

I am not sure how the last group of believers can resolve these contradictory statements/empirical findings (e.g., ADHD is underdiagnosed, its rates are stable, and yet national surveys indicate over 20% prevalence among teenage boys), but with your permission, I would like to raise a disturbing 'either-way' enigma: If the *DSM* is wrong and the actual rates of ADHD are not 3–5%, but 9.6–13.6% [15], or even higher, as documented in this chapter, what can explain this huge rise in ADHD rates within a short period of 40 years, since the first introduction of the disorder in *DSM*-III? This is an evolutionary miracle. At the same time, if the *DSM* is right, and 'only' 5% of children are eligible for the diagnosis of ADHD, then about 5–15% of all children are unjustifiably diagnosed, at least in some places. In other words, for every single true-positive diagnosis, clinicians make approximately two false-positive errors (and this is before calculating the false-negative errors of the proclaimed underdiagnosed cases).

As mentioned earlier, in my view, the conservative *DSM* estimate of 5% that is suggested in this second option is too large to be considered deviant (see Figure 1). However, even if we are willing to accept the 5% estimate as an indication for a deviant behavior, we are still facing massive rates of unjustified overdiagnoses — millions of false diagnoses that extend far beyond the correct ones, according to the *DSM*. In my opinion, even faithful believers of the disorder should be worried, as the 'father of ADHD' (see the Introduction), Dr. Conners himself said: "the numbers make it look like an epidemic… well, it's not. It's preposterous" [38]. How come we have reached a point where the overdiagnosis problem is significantly larger than the correct diagnoses? Are so many clinicians making inappropriate diagnoses? And if they do, how do the few 'super' clinicians that manage to make the right diagnosis accomplish this complicated task? What helps them differentiate between real and unreal

ADHD? The *DSM* alone does not provide tools to make this differential diagnosis.

I have actually sent some of these questions to the editor-in-chief of the *Journal of Attention Disorders* — the acknowledgeable academic home for ADHD research — after he explicitly admitted (as part of our correspondence regarding a data-availability issue discussed in Chapter 12) that "at times, zealous efforts" are made "to pathologize normal, developmental variations in children" [39], however these questions were not answered. One might think that overdiagnosis is a small price to pay compared with the advantages of correct diagnoses. This claim might have been valid if the overdiagnosis problem was marginal compared to the main phenomenon. However, as shown above, this is not the case at all.

Even if there is a small percentage of children that could have fit this hypothetical *DSM* condition, the fact that most children are diagnosed unjustifiably is sufficient, in my view, to stop using the clinical label of ADHD. In other words, believers of the theoretical construct called ADHD, who are also warning from overdiagnosis and overtreatment [8], should acknowledge, in my view, that the original term of ADHD has lost its meaning, as so many children are being called 'ADHD children', even though they have no brain dysregulations whatsoever. Assuming that most clinicians do their best to provide the most accurate diagnosis to their patients, the overdiagnosis spotlight should be directed at the very diagnostic instructions they receive — that is the current *DSM* criteria, which apparently are not sufficient to make a reliable diagnosis.

Alternatively, if the first option is correct and ADHD rates did rise to fantastic levels of 13%, and over 20% (at least among some populations), then I hope that even the most devout believers of the disorder would agree that ADHD does not meet the basic diagnostic criterion of deviance. After all, if such a large number of children have ADHD, it begs the question: who is abnormal, the children or us, the adults who are diagnosing them?

Taken together, the large number of real clinical errors, the epidemic-like rise in the reported rates of ADHD, and the instability of the diagnosis over time and across populations (i.e., the strong dependency of this biomedical brain disorder on multiple sociodemographic variables, such as age, gender, and religious affiliation), all indicate that the theoretical construct of ADHD suffers from an extremely poor scientific reliability (see also Table 4 at the General Discussion). Without decent levels of reliability, clinicians and scientists are essentially unable to accurately determine which children really suffer from ADHD, and the entire scientific tower of the diagnosis collapses.

References

1. Mohammadi, M.-R., *et al.*, *Prevalence of ADHD and its comorbidities in a population-based sample.* Journal of Attention Disorders, 2021. **25**(8): p. 1058–1067.
2. Joshi, H.M. and M. Angolkar, *Prevalence of ADHD in primary school children in Belagavi City, India.* Journal of Attention Disorders, 2021. **25**(2): p. 154–160.
3. Sandstrom, A., *et al.*, *Prevalence of attention-deficit/hyperactivity disorder in people with mood disorders: A systematic review and meta-analysis.* Acta Psychiatrica Scandinavica, 2021. **143**(5): p. 380–391.
4. Wong, A.W.W.A. and S.D. Landes, *Expanding Understanding of Racial-Ethnic Differences in ADHD Prevalence Rates among Children to Include Asians and Alaskan Natives/American Indians.* Journal of Attention Disorders, 2021: p. 10870547211027932.
5. APA, *Diagnostic and Statistical Manual of Mental Disorders (DSM-5®).* 2013: American Psychiatric Association.
6. Barkley, R.A. and M. Fischer, *The Milwaukee Longitudinal Study of Hyperactive (ADHD) Children*, in *Attention Deficit Hyperactivity Disorder: Adult Outcome and Its Predictors.* 2017, Oxford University Press. p. 63–104.
7. Davidovitch, M., *et al.*, *Age-Specific Time Trends in Incidence Rates of Autism Spectrum Disorder Following Adaptation of DSM-5 and Other ASD-Related Regulatory Changes in Israel.* Autism Research, 2020. **13**(11): p. 1893–1901.

8. Davidovitch, M., *et al.*, *Diagnosis despite clinical ambiguity: physicians' perspectives on the rise in Autism Spectrum disorder incidence.* BMC Psychiatry, 2021. **21**(1): p. 150.
9. Polanczyk, G., *et al.*, *The worldwide prevalence of ADHD: a systematic review and metaregression analysis.* American journal of psychiatry, 2007. **164**(6): p. 942–948.
10. Kooij, J.J.S., *et al.*, *Updated European Consensus Statement on diagnosis and treatment of adult ADHD.* European Psychiatry, 2019. **56**: p. 14–34.
11. Vos, T., *et al.*, *Global, regional, and national incidence, prevalence, and years lived with disability for 328 diseases and injuries for 195 countries, 1990–2016: a systematic analysis for the Global Burden of Disease Study 2016.* The Lancet, 2017. **390**(10100): p. 1211–1259.
12. Polanczyk, G.V., *et al.*, *Annual Research Review: A meta-analysis of the worldwide prevalence of mental disorders in children and adolescents.* Journal of Child Psychology and Psychiatry, 2015. **56**(3): p. 345–365.
13. APA, *Diagnostic and Statistical Manual of Mental Disorders - Third Edition (DSM-III).* 1980: American Psychiatric Association (APA).
14. Visser, S.N., *et al.*, *Trends in the parent-report of health care provider-diagnosed and medicated attention-deficit/hyperactivity disorder: United States, 2003–2011.* Journal of the American Academy of Child & Adolescent Psychiatry, 2014. **53**(1): p. 34–46.
15. Danielson, M.L., et al., *Prevalence of Parent-Reported ADHD Diagnosis and Associated Treatment Among U.S. Children and Adolescents, 2016.* Journal of Clinical Child & Adolescent Psychology, 2018. **47**(2): p. 199–212.
16. Biederman, J. and T. Spencer, *Attention-deficit/hyperactivity disorder (ADHD) as a noradrenergic disorder.* Biological Psychiatry, 1999. **46**(9): p. 1234–1242.
17. Awadalla, N.J., *et al.*, *Role of school teachers in identifying attention deficit hyperactivity disorder among primary school children in Mansoura, Egypt.* EMHJ-Eastern Mediterranean Health Journal, 2016. **22**(8): p. 586–595.
18. Pineda, D.A., *et al.*, *Confirmation of the high prevalence of attention deficit disorder in a Colombian community.* Revista de Neurologia, 2001. **32**(3): p. 217–222.

19. Safavi, P., F. Ganji, and A. Bidad, *Prevalence of attention-deficit hyperactivity disorder in students and needs modification of mental health services in Shahrekord, Iran in 2013.* Journal of Clinical and Diagnostic Research: JCDR, 2016. **10**(4): p. LC25.
20. Baumgaertel, A., M.L. Wolraich, and M. Dietrich, *Comparison of diagnostic criteria for attention deficit disorders in a German elementary school sample.* Journal of the American Academy of Child & Adolescent Psychiatry, 1995. **34**(5): p. 629–638.
21. Guardiola, A., F.D. Fuchs, and N.T. Rotta, *Prevalence of attention-deficit hyperactivity disorders in students: comparison between DSM-IV and neuropsychological criteria.* Arquivos de Neuro-psiquiatria, 2000. **58**: p. 401–407.
22. Gadow, K.D., *et al.*, *Comparison of attention-deficit/hyperactivity disorder symptom subtypes in Ukrainian school children.* Journal of the American Academy of Child & Adolescent Psychiatry, 2000. **39**(12): p. 1520–1527.
23. Merzon, E., *et al.*, *ADHD as a Risk Factor for Infection With Covid-19.* Journal of Attention Disorders, 2020. **25**(13): p. 1783–1790.
24. Ophir, Y., *Evidence that the Diagnosis of ADHD Does Not Reflect a Chronic Bio-Medical Disease.* Ethical Human Psychology and Psychiatry, 2022. **23–2**.
25. Ra, C.K., *et al.*, *Association of Digital Media Use With Subsequent Symptoms of Attention-Deficit/Hyperactivity Disorder Among Adolescents.* JAMA, 2018. **320**(3): p. 255–263.
26. Ophir, Y., *et al.*, *The turker blues: Hidden factors behind increased depression rates among Amazon's Mechanical Turkers.* Clinical Psychological Science, 2020. **8**(1): p. 65–83.
27. Kessler, R.C., *et al.*, *The World Health Organization Adult ADHD Self-Report Scale (ASRS): a short screening scale for use in the general population.* Psychological Medicine, 2005. **35**(2): p. 245–256.
28. International Narcotics Control Board, *Psychotropic Substances Statistics for 2018 Assessments of Annual Medical and Scientific Requirements.* 2019, https://www.incb.org/documents/Psychotropics/technical-publications/2019/PSY_Technical_Publication_2019.pdf: United Nations - Vienna.

29. Smith, M., *Hyperactive: The controversial history of ADHD.* 2013: Reaktion books.
30. Smith, M., *Hyperactive Around the World? The History of ADHD in Global Perspective.* Social History of Medicine, 2017. **30**(4): p. 767–787.
31. Timimi, S. and E. Taylor, *ADHD is best understood as a cultural construct.* British Journal of Psychiatry, 2004. **184**(1): p. 8–9.
32. Bergey, M.R., *et al.*, *Global perspectives on ADHD: social dimensions of diagnosis and treatment in sixteen countries.* 2018: JHU Press.
33. Li, K., *Religion and medicalization: The case of ADHD.* Journal for the Scientific Study of Religion, 2013. **52**(2): p. 309–327.
34. Paulus, M.P., *et al.*, *Screen media activity and brain structure in youth: Evidence for diverse structural correlation networks from the ABCD study.* Neuroimage, 2019. **185**: p. 140–153.
35. Bolotnyy, V. and N. Emanuel, *Why do women earn less than men? Evidence from bus and train operators.* 2018.
36. Sayal, K., *et al.*, *ADHD in children and young people: prevalence, care pathways, and service provision.* The Lancet Psychiatry, 2018. **5**(2): p. 175–186.
37. Bolea-Alamañac, B., *et al.*, *Evidence-based guidelines for the pharmacological management of attention deficit hyperactivity disorder: Update on recommendations from the British Association for Psychopharmacology.* Journal of Psychopharmacology, 2014. **28**(3): p. 179–203.
38. Schwarz, A., *The selling of attention deficit disorder.* New York Times, 2013. **14**.
39. Ophir, Y. and Y. Shir-Raz, *Discrepancies in Studies on ADHD and COVID-19 Raise Concerns Regarding the Risks of Stimulant Treatments During an Active Pandemic.* Accepted Manuscript. Ethical Human Psychology and Psychiatry.

“

“I have great news for you… Jeremy… You have an amazing brain. Your brain is incredible… Your brain is like a Ferrari race-car engine… But there is one problem… You have bicycle brakes. Your brakes are not strong enough to control the powerful brain you've got… But don't worry. I am a brake specialist. I will help you strengthen your brakes.”

Hallowell, E. (2021). *Your Brain Is a Ferrari.* Retrieved in November, 2021 from ADDitude's website [1]

Chapter 3
Does ADHD meet the criterion of Dysfunction?

The diabetes metaphor, which was presented in the Introduction of this book to illustrate the biomedical consensus regarding Attention Deficit Hyperactivity Disorder (ADHD), is sometimes replaced by less disturbing similes, such as the "bicycle brakes" by Dr. Edward Hallowell. When talking to children, Dr. Hallowell, another influential authority in the field of ADHD, recommends the readership of ADDitude (a highly popular information source about ADHD) to begin with the child's strengths ("your brain is like a Ferrari") and only then move to describe her/his brain deficit ("you have bicycle brakes"). This communication tactic probably has some value for some children. However, it still holds the same biological deterministic message, something along the following lines: You have a chronic brain problem that could cause you a lot of trouble throughout your life. It has nothing to do with school setting or academic functioning. You were born with a brain deficit, which should be managed medically [2, 3]. You therefore need a "brake specialist" physician that could prescribe you the appropriate treatment of choice (Introduction) that will "strengthen" (but not 'fix') your impaired "brain brakes".

But how do these impaired "brain brakes" look like in the real world? After all, they are not really detectable through neuroimaging measures (Chapter 6). To answer this question, we should inspect the behavioral indications of this alleged brain deficit, as they are described in the *Diagnostic and Statistical Manual of Mental Disorders* (*DSM*). Surprisingly, the entire list of 18 symptoms of ADHD addresses only one of the "Four Ds" criteria of psychiatric diagnosis — the criterion of Dysfunction (e.g., "often has difficulty organizing tasks"). In other words, none of the listed symptoms reflect the other negative dimensions of mental disorders, that of Distress or Danger. Without these dimensions and without convincing evidence that ADHD is a Deviant phenomenon (Chapter 2), special attention should therefore be given to the validity of the Dysfunction criterion in ADHD, that is to the question: To what extent does ADHD cause significant and substantial impairment in everyday functioning (regardless of school-related demands)?

The dysfunction criterion in neurodevelopmental disorders

To answer this underlying question of the current chapter, we first need to define what "significant impairment in everyday functioning" entails. A simple definition for impairment in functioning can be extracted from common clinical assessment tools that aim to evaluate the individual's ability to perform mundane activities of daily living, such as getting dressed, taking a shower, and cleaning oneself after using the toilet [e.g., 4]. These basic daily practices may be impaired, for example, in severe cases of Autism Spectrum Disorder or Intellectual Disability — the neighboring *DSM* disorders that share the same neurodevelopmental clustering with ADHD. Of course, dysfunctions in mental disorders are not always so pervasive, but then, other fundamental criterions are involved, such as distress or danger. Individuals with Major Depressive Disorder, for example, may maintain their ability to go to work and take out the trash, but their distressed emotions and dangerous suicidal thoughts — two hallmarks of the disorder [5] — allow them to be eligible for a mental health diagnosis. As mentioned in Chapter 1, there is a trade-off between the four criteria of psychiatric diagnosis. Thus, if we wish to diagnose a person based on the dysfunction criterion only, the impact of this criterion should be pervasive.

The centrality of the dysfunction criterion in neurodevelopmental disorders, the cluster of disorders that includes ADHD, can be learnt from the *DSM* itself. The checklist of symptoms in multiple disorders is usually followed by an explicit requirement that the symptoms will cause significant impairments in daily functioning; otherwise, they may not be sufficient for making the neuropsychiatric diagnosis. In Autism Spectrum Disorder for example, the *DSM* requires that the symptoms will "cause clinically significant impairment in social, occupational, or other important areas of current functioning" [5, p. 50]. In Intellectual Disability, the functioning deficits should "result in failure to meet developmental and sociocultural standards for personal independence and social responsibility" and the person with the disability typically cannot perform simple daily activities "without ongoing support" (p. 33). Deviant, low levels of intelligence alone, as explained in Chapter 2, are not enough to make the diagnosis. The *DSM* determines that the poor intelligence characterizing the disorder must be manifested in the person's daily functioning. In ADHD however, the dysfunction criterion appears in a completely different form.

The strange softening of the dysfunction criterion

The short history of ADHD teaches that ADHD is an ever-changing concept [6, 7]. Aside from this reliability problem, it seems that "as time goes by", the behaviors thought to be indicative of the disorder are becoming less and less disruptive. Proponents of the disorder who insist that its first record preceded the discovery of the marvels — amphetamines (1937) and methylphenidate (1963) — and appeared in the 100-year-old lecture (1902) by Sir George Still, know all too well that Still described "an abnormal defect of ethical control in children", which included serious behavioral disruptions, such as cruel brutality and abuse of animals [8]. This serious "moral defect" is, of course, no longer part of the ADHD diagnosis. However, there are indications that the modern formulation of ADHD — the one from the third edition of the *DSM* (1980), which was the first to present the term 'attention' — still comprised relatively serious behavioral impairments.

Back in 1979 for example, when Barkley initiated the Milwaukee longitudinal study (for further information, see further in this chapter), he assigned children to the experimental group of the study only if their symptoms were at the extreme end of the normal distribution (at least 2 Standard Deviation points above the mean) and only if they had pervasive behavioral problems at home. Importantly, these behaviors had to be observed outside of school during mundane activities at home, such as: getting dressed, bathing, and playing [9].

Correspondingly, the diagnostic criteria of the fourth edition of the *DSM*, which was published in 1994, specifically determined that: "there must be clear evidence of clinically significant impairment in social, academic, or occupational functioning" [10, p. 84].

It was only in 2013 that something really strange happened. For some reason (see Chapter 12), the authors of the contemporary edition of the psychiatric manual (*DSM*-5) conducted a subtle, yet dramatic modification of the "significant impairment" requirement. According to the updated manual, a diagnosis of ADHD can be given when there is "clear evidence that the symptoms *interfere* with, or *reduce* the quality of, social, academic, or occupational functioning" [5, p. 60]. For an outsider, this modified wording may seem like a minor semantic difference. However, this difference represents a major change in the very definition of the disorder — especially considering the fact that the entire diagnostic tower of ADHD is made out of dysfunction-related bricks only.

I will not be surprised if this softened criterion of 'reduction in functioning' contributed to the rise in ADHD rates described in Chapter 2. A cohort study conducted among a large representative sample of young adults, for example, revealed that the application of the *DSM*-5 diagnostic criteria yielded a 27% increase in ADHD rates, compared with the rates obtained using the previous *DSM*-IV criteria [11]. In a way, a softened criterion of dysfunction is like a magic wand in a game of rock paper scissors. It beats them all. Partially reduced functionality in specific daily tasks is part of being human. A person (myself, don't tell anyone) who has difficulties in spatial perception will experience reduced ability to park the car in reverse or to find his way back to the conference hotel, when travelling. A child who tends to introversion will probably experience reduced levels of social functioning in the classroom and a child who is usually off-key will experience reduced levels of functioning in the school choir. Therefore, to make a psychiatric diagnosis, it is not sufficient to demonstrate an interference or reduction in functioning. The person should experience *clinically significant and pervasive impairment* in multiple daily functioning (see also Chapter 1).

The vague and subjective threshold for dysfunction

Not only does the modified dysfunction requirement have very little diagnostic value, the way that the *DSM* phrases the actual symptoms of the disorder also suggests that children can be eligible for the diagnosis even when they do not suffer a substantiative dysfunction. Most of the symptoms reflect minor behavioral difficulties (e.g., "difficulty keeping materials and belongings in order") that usually improve with age (see further in this chapter). In fact, the *DSM* specifically allows clinicians to diagnose a child with a "mild" form of the disorder, in which the "symptoms result in no more than minor impairments in social or occupational functioning" [5, p. 60]. Let me repeat this shocking piece of information: A child can be diagnosed with a 'real' biogenetic psychiatric disorder that is typically treated with psychoactive drugs, even though none of the required Four Ds criteria really exist.

Recently, this problem of softened (and almost meaningless) criterion of dysfunction has been manifested in empirical research. A large study from Denmark that targeted this issue failed to demonstrate an explicit threshold for impairment in dysfunction in ADHD [12]. According to the authors, "there was no clear evidence for a discrete, nonarbitrary symptom severity threshold with regard to impairment" (p. 1). Readers who are familiar with the *DSM* are probably not surprised to learn about this finding. The phrasing of all the 18 symptoms mentioned in the *DSM* opens with the word "often" (e.g., "often loses things"). But how much exactly is "often"? Without the need to demonstrate clear evidence for impairment, the diagnostic mission becomes highly subjective and vague (perhaps this vagueness could explain the prevalence gaps described in Chapter 2). Consider for example the following six representative symptoms that, if they exist, could be indicative of a predominantly hyperactive/impulsive presentation of ADHD: (1) "Often leaves seat in situations when remaining seated is expected"; (2) "Often runs about or climbs in situations where it is not appropriate"; (3) "Often unable to play or engage in leisure activities quietly"; (4) "Often talks excessively"; (5) "Often blurts out an answer before a question has been completed"; and (6) "Often has trouble waiting his or her turn" [5, p. 60]. Since almost every child in the world may experience some level of these (childish) behaviors, it is crucial that we set a clear cut-off point for the word "often."

Indeed, various ADHD scales were developed for this exact purpose of quantifying the intensity of these childish behaviors, but again, without a rigid criterion of impairment in dysfunction, the classification of these behaviors relies only on the criterion of deviance — a criterion that is not met in ADHD, as shown in Chapter 2. Moreover, these scales typically suffer from poor reliability. Teachers provide different ratings from parents and mothers provide different ratings from fathers [13, 14]. Finally, there is a large overlap between the potential symptoms of ADHD. A child who "often runs about" is also a child that is "often unable to take part in quiet activities" and "often leaves seat". Similarly, a child who "often blurts out an answer" is also likely to be evaluated as a child who "often talks excessively" and often "has trouble waiting his or her turn." To some extent, the aforementioned six symptoms can be seen as an artificial expansion of only two core behaviors.

The suspicious tailoring of the criterion to school settings

These basic reliability gaps are exacerbated when considering the intertwined relationships that exist between the symptoms of the disorder and the external demands of school environments. Where do children "blurt out an answer before a question has been completed"? Where are children expected to "remain seated" for lengthy periods of time? The answer to these rhetoric questions is that, not only does the phrasing of the symptoms reflect minor dysfunctions, these dysfunctions also appear predominantly in school. The *DSM* itself states multiple examples for dysfunctions at school settings. Representative examples from the *inattention* cluster of symptoms are: "makes careless mistakes in schoolwork", "has difficulty remaining focused during lectures… or lengthy reading", "fails to finish schoolwork", "dislikes tasks that require sustained mental effort… schoolwork or homework", and "loses things… school materials, pencils, books, tools, wallets, keys, paperwork" [5, p. 59].

Indeed, the authors of the *DSM* seem to recognize this problematic reliance on school environment/demands, which undermines the conceptualization of the disorder as a pervasive biogenetic brain deficit. They specifically added a constraint to the diagnosis, according to which "*several* inattentive or hyperactive-impulsive symptoms" should be present "in *two* or more settings" (p. 60); that is, in at least one setting outside of school. But this reservation is in fact another example for an artificial modification of an earlier, more rigid *DSM* criterion, according to which the *impairment* from the symptoms should have been present in at least two settings [15]. Today, the *DSM*-based convention is that the life-disturbing impairment or the full presentation of the disorder do not need to be evident independently, outside of school context. In the current edition of the manual, once children demonstrate two mild ADHD-related behaviors at home (assuming that the phrase "several symptoms" means at least two symptoms), in addition to their difficulties at school, such as 'talking excessively' or 'running around', they can be eligible for a clinical diagnosis of ADHD.

The astounding fact that ADHD can exist despite its selective disappearance outside of school premises is explicitly acknowledged in the apologetic, and in my opinion, mind-blowing *DSM* rationalization, according to which: "signs of the disorder may be minimal or absent when the individual is receiving frequent rewards for appropriate behavior, is under close supervision, is in a novel setting, is engaged in especially interesting activities, has consistent external stimulation (e.g., via electronic screens), or is interacting in one-on-one situations (e.g., the clinician's office)" [5, p. 61]. In other words, despite the notion that this chronic and pervasive brain disorder affects all aspects of life, it may be quite illusive outside of mainstream school settings. Miraculously, the innate difficulty to sustain attention can disappear when the child engages in interesting activities, including purely attention-based activities, such as reading books (I personally witnessed this miracle with ADHD 3rd graders who read the entire book series of Harry Potter and The Adventures of Captain Underpants). The problem with this rationalization is that it allows the existence of an absurd and ethically disturbing medical situation. Clinicians can now diagnose children with ADHD even if they do not observe the symptoms directly, since the symptoms can disappear when the child is "interacting in one-on-one situations (e.g., the clinician's office)" — note that the parenthesis with the clinician's office example is stated by the authors of the *DSM* themselves. De facto, clinicians can rely on questionnaires and testimonials from parents and teachers who report relatively benign dysfunctions, such as mistakes in schoolwork, a messy backpack, or fidgeting in one's seat as solid indicators for the existence of a neurodevelopmental disorder.

The frequent disappearance of the dysfunctions

Aside from the ethical issue, we must ask how it is possible that individuals with an objective deficit in sustained attention can maintain attention for such prolonged periods, sometimes in a strenuous cognitive effort to solve a complex puzzle or to break a personal record? A popular answer, which seems to be more widespread in the general media than in the scientific discourse, is that individuals with ADHD tend to engage in more hyperfocus experiences [16], where they 'live in the zone' or 'fixate like a laser' on topics of interests (even when these interests demand high cognitive effort). Beside the facts that hyperfocus is not listed as an official symptom of ADHD and has not achieved sufficient empirical support, as shown in a recent study that did not demonstrate differences in hyperfocus experiences between individuals with and without ADHD [17], the hyperfocus argument, once again, undermines the very conceptualization of the disorder as an "Attention Deficit".

The reality is that most life experiences and activities require some levels of sustained attention and cognitive control, whether in school settings or outside of school settings. Attention is a required condition for any human awareness, and it is needed for all human activities, including the ones that are usually held outside of school settings, such as a highly arousing, Ninja obstacle course competition (a preferred activity among children with a predominant hyperactive/impulsive presentation of ADHD), or a more relaxed, arts and crafts workshop (a preferred activity among children with a predominant inattention presentation of ADHD). In fact, activities that are characterized with high levels of attention, the ones that were named 'hyperfocus experiences' earlier, are more likely to appear outside of educational settings [17]. Perhaps this could explain why diagnosed children can excel in complex tasks that require high cognitive control and behavioral inhibition, such as video games, just as much as their undiagnosed peers [18]. In fact, certain action-oriented video games are now being studied as a potential platform for enhancing cognitive control [19, 20]. It seems that once the 'boring element' is removed from the cognitive task, the executive functions of ADHD-type individuals operate adequately. A study, for example, that used a modified Computerized Performance Test (CPT), which included the traditional cognitive-control tasks (see Chapters 1 and 6), but also an engaging and fast-paced play environment, showed that the expected performance differences between adults with and without ADHD evaporate when the cognitive task is held in a stimulating environment [21]. In other words, the 'problem' in ADHD may be motivational (rather than a pure deficit in executive functioning), consisting mainly of a strong reluctance to be bored.

But when they are not bored (remember the arts and crafts example), and when they are highly motivated (remember the Ninja example), diagnosed children can reach great achievements even in fields that require superb cognitive control. It is usually easier to notice these achievements when they grow up, when their latitude to choose their preferred daily environment is increased [22]. For example, studies conducted in highly stimulating environments, such as in combat military contexts, found that the functioning levels of adults with ADHD were equivalent to, and sometimes higher than, the functioning levels of adults without ADHD [23, 24]. In some cases, adults with ADHD can even reach spectacular achievements. All-time Olympic champion Michael Phelps had to recruit all his cognitive resources to produce the most precise swimming movements, without any errors [25]. All-time best basketball player (yes, even better than LeBron), Michael Jordan, had to stay sharp as a knife, in front of thousands of shouting people who try to distract him during free throws [26]. Even Leonardo da Vinci, who is suspected to have had severe ADHD, which disabled him from completing most of his artworks, managed eventually to create masterpieces like the Last Supper and the Mona Lisa [27].

Of course, most children with ADHD will not become Olympic medalists, but many of them could easily function in multiple everyday environments, such as the tough business world or the competitive media market. On the positive side of ADHD, psychiatrist Dale Archer lists multiple traits that could become the diagnosed person's greatest strengths, including the abilities to think out-of-the-box in a non-linear manner, work effectively under external pressures, overcome downfalls, and engage in multitasking activities [28]. He even offers a simple conceptualization, according to which ADHD can be seen as a tendency to have a very low boredom threshold. Indeed, this low threshold probably constrains children's ability to concentrate at school; however, it can also increase their ability to reach novel ideas and insights [29–31]. Thus, together, with their energetic and spirited character, ADHD type individuals can excel in multiple settings and perform well in various situations (see Chapters 4 and 5 for theory-driven descriptions of the bright side of ADHD).

The puzzling selective use of medications

But even if we disregard all the evidence regarding the positive aspects of ADHD, real-life observations suggest, as claimed earlier, that the essential dysfunctions that are associated with ADHD appear mainly in school. In my own research on the biomedical perception of ADHD (see Chapter 2), I 'discovered' a well-known truth: the pharmacological treatment for ADHD that should be taken continuously to cope with the wide-ranging implications of this chronic brain deficit, is used almost exclusively for the improvement of school-related behaviors and performances [32]. Prescribed stimulant medications, in my research, were mostly used during high school age and between the ages 23–24, which are usually the ages of undergraduate students in Israel. Most users of the medications discontinued their treatment plan after several months, and almost all users did not use the medications during weekends and holidays. The users in my study were very open and honest regarding their motives for using the medications. Almost all participants used the medications to improve their academic performance in school (55.6%) or in college/professional studies (39.1%). Medications were very rarely used for managing other aspects of life, such as emotional or social functioning, which are said to be affected by this neurodevelopmental deficit [33]. This gap between the implied, biomedical perception of the physicians prescribing the 'treatment of choice' for ADHD and the actual medication-related practices of patients suggests that the alleged dysfunctions associated with ADHD are confined mainly to school-related demands.

Similar conclusions were derived from my COVID-19 study that focused on children (see Chapter 2). On the one hand, almost all diagnosed children were given prescriptions for ADHD medications by their physicians. On the other hand, and in a sharp contrast to the implied biomedical notions of the physicians prescribing the medications (see the Introduction), most of the parents in the study decided to discontinue their children's medication treatment during the COVID lockdown. From the parents' perspective: "there is no need to take medications when there is no school" [32]. This finding received unexpected support from the large COVID-19 study that investigated thousands of medical records in Israel (see Chapters 2 and 12). This study revealed (unintentionally) that only a quarter of the diagnosed individuals (24.6%) purchased at least three consecutive ADHD-medication-prescriptions during the 12 months that preceded the study [34]. Together, these studies suggest that most parents do not believe that their children's daily dysfunctions require a constant pharmacological management. They associate these dysfunctions instead with school-related demands.

Regrettably, my last study on children during the COVID-19 also revealed a concerning phenomenon, according to which some parents (who are probably encouraged by physicians and school teachers) exercise their authority to convince their children to take their medications during school days, despite their children's persistent objection and despite the adverse side-effects they had experienced [32]. Of course, if the medications are necessary to manage a dangerous and harmful condition, as suggested by the biomedical approach, then these daily battles may be justified. However, here we see that, in most cases, this problematic daily interaction between parents and children is fueled by the parental concern that their child's performance/behavior in school will be impaired. Without this concern, when school demands are taken out of the equation, the child's voice and personal needs can finally be heard.

The 'healing' power of age

Not only do the dysfunctions associated with ADHD tend to disappear outside of the school context, they also seem to be attenuated over time, when the child becomes an adult. As discussed in Chapter 2, the age factor plays a significant role in the fluctuating prevalence of ADHD. The 2016 national survey of the Centers for Disease Control and Prevention (CDC) documented a linear increase in lifetime diagnosis of ADHD among children [35], starting with 2.4% among 2–5-year-old children (approximately 388,000 children), 9.6% among 6–11-year-old- school aged children (2.4 million), and 13.6% among 12–17-year-old adolescents (3.3 million). Then, miraculously, the prevalence of ADHD drops abruptly during adulthood.

This strange drop is also evident in the *DSM* itself. Despite the alleged consensus that ADHD is a lifelong neurological condition [33], the *DSM* acknowledges a large prevalence gap in ADHD rates between children (5%) and adults (2.5%) [5]. Surprisingly, in contrast to the clinical course of many other mental disorders, a spontaneous recovery seems to occur among at least half of the adults who suffered from this "brain disorder" as children (at school). Similarly, findings from Barkley's Milwaukee Longitudinal Study mentioned before showed that at least 36% of the hyperactive children participating in the study had fully recovered as adults [9]. In fact, when the researchers of this influential study used the original *DSM*-IV criteria for ADHD alongside the required functional impairment criterion, a total of 76% (!) did not meet the clinical threshold for ADHD. This finding is particularly noteworthy in light of the fact that the original experimental group of hyperactive children was very carefully constructed in this study, using rigorous criteria of 2 standard deviations above the mean level of symptoms and pervasive daily behavioral problems at home [9].

The age gap in the prevalence rates of the disorder is sometimes rationalized by proponents of the disorder as a sign for a partial remission (but not disappearance) of the symptoms during adulthood, which makes the disorder harder to detect. From their perspective, adult ADHD is, in fact, underdiagnosed [33], and its 'real' prevalence should be similar to the prevalence of the disorder among children. This is because, ADHD in their view, and as mentioned in the Introduction of this book, is "a neurodevelopmental and heritable disorder with a lifespan perspective: starting in childhood, persisting in adulthood until old age" [33, p. 27].

To investigate this claim regarding the chronic nature of the diagnosis (i.e., the stability of the diagnosis within the individual), I have asked adult participants with and without a former diagnosis of ADHD, to complete the Adult ADHD Self-Report Scale (ASRS) — a highly used screening tool that has been approved by the World Health Organization [36]. I have then calculated the percentage of false classifications of the Adult ADHD scale and revealed that the **majority** of the formerly diagnosed participants (56.6%) were not eligible for the diagnosis, according to their scores on the Adult ADHD Scale [32]. In other words, these adults did not exhibit severe symptoms that impaired their daily functioning, in a complete contrast to the implied assumptions of the neurogenetic perception of ADHD as a lifelong deficit. Indeed, one might argue that the accuracy of the Adult Scale is not perfect to begin with. However, this figure represents a significantly higher false-negative rate than the 31.3% rate that was expected, according to the reported sensitivity scores of the original scale, $\chi^2 = 20.34$, $p < 0.001$. Interestingly, on the other side of this unreliable coin, a total of 9.5% of the non-diagnosed individuals actually did meet the ASRS criterion for ADHD. This figure represents a significantly higher false-positive rate than the 0.5% rate that was expected according to the reported specificity scores of the original scale, $\chi^2 = 911.77$, $p < 0.001$. Altogether, these findings suggest that the reliability of the diagnosis is unstable also at the intra-individual level (i.e., not only between groups, as discussed in Chapter 2), thus undermining the notion that ADHD is a lifelong condition.

Another empirical support to the 'healing power of age' has emerged in the seminal longitudinal Randomized Control Trial (RCT) conducted by the National Institute of Mental Health (NIMH), which was called the 'Multimodal Treatment of ADHD' study (for more details, see Chapter 9). Three years after the initiation of this high-quality RCT, the researchers admitted honestly that they were "struck by the remarkable degree of improvement in all four groups... in symptoms and overall functioning... This degree of improvement found in all of the subjects over time, regardless of which treatment these children received, may not have received sufficient attention in the previous treatment research literature... Such changes... may reflect a natural waning of symptoms..." [37, pp. 998–999].

The impact of the individuals' age on the severity of the symptoms and the overall functioning of the child is, in my view, a central characteristic of ADHD that might help us uncover a simple, yet somewhat hidden truth: Children grow up! Throughout life, and especially during childhood and adolescence, the human brain develops, adapts, and improves in accordance with the changing needs of reality [38, 39]. Even those who strongly believe that ADHD is a real medical disorder admit that, in some cases, the dysfunctions associated with ADHD are simply a reflection of the developmental stage of the child. Otherwise, how can they explain the fact that in most Western-oriented countries, there is a greater prevalence of diagnoses and treatments among children who are younger than the majority of their classmates [40–42]? This consistent finding in the literature suggests that teachers and clinicians tend to confuse children's immaturity with a chronic mental health disability.

This confusion between immaturity and ADHD is not only relevant to children who are younger than their classmates. The pace of children's physical and mental development varies from child to child and some children are bound to be slower to develop than others. This does not mean that they have a brain deficit. On the contrary, the common developmental ground of all children (except perhaps from children with severe impairments, such as Intellectual Disability) is that they will continue to acquire multiple cognitive and behavioral skills as they develop. The brain development that occurs during childhood and adolescence is immense: hyperactive behaviors are mitigated and cognitive executive functions become more sophisticated [43], especially when the child grows up in a loving and supportive environment. Adults, by definition, are less hyperactive and more settled, than children. This of course, does not mean that adults cannot behave impulsively or be easily distracted, but they too, were probably more impulsive and more inattentive when they were children. A large study, for example, which investigated over 10,000 participants, found that the ability to sustain attention (as measured in discrimination performance and response time consistency) increases rapidly between the ages of 10–16 and continues to increase, though at a more modest pace, between the ages of 17–43 [44]. These findings challenge the basic biomedical assumption, as if the ADHD child has an objective brain deficit in cognitive executive functions because these cognitive functions are yet to be developed and improved. Moreover, even if one day, brain differences will be used as biological markers for poor cognitive abilities, they might simply reflect different developmental paces of children and they are probably going to disappear, once the child's brain completes its development (for a further discussion of this point, see Chapter 6).

A different outlook on children's dysfunctions

All in all, the evidence brought in this chapter shows that the dysfunction criterion is not met in the case of ADHD, at least not objectively. The dysfunctions associated with the disorder are unreliable and, unfortunately, seem to be tailored by leaders of the field specifically and artificially to school behaviors. An alternative, and in my opinion more reasonable, explanation for the labeling of children with neuropsychiatric conditions is that normative and age-appropriate behaviors of children (e.g., "often fails to finish schoolwork", "often runs about or climbs") are being medicalized unjustifiably, mainly in response to school-related demands [45, 46]. As well-articulated by Dr. Thomas Armstrong, a leading critic of the disorder (see the Introduction), "we don't let kids be kids anymore" [47; Chapter 4, Reason #1].

The developmental period of childhood, in most cultures, is viewed as a wonderful time of physical activity, play, unruly behavior, and even disobedience and irritability towards adult caregivers [48]. These behaviors characterize the young of many mammalian species, yet they are prohibited for children in schools. Using the wording of the *DSM*, it is not hard to imagine how stereotypical childish behaviors such as running around, fist-fighting, making a mess, and bravely engaging in adventurous and risky activities, are quickly turning into medical symptoms such as: "often runs about or climbs in situations **where it is inappropriate**" or "often leaves seat in situations **when remaining seated is expected**" [5, p.60, bold added by Y.O.], especially in school settings where these behaviors are indeed considered inappropriate. But once again, are we allowed to conceptualize these mild, age-appropriate, and sometimes even funny or mischievous dysfunctions, as a lifelong brain deficit, and dare to treat them with powerful medications? The answer to this question, as shown here, is quite straightforward in my opinion, but the following chapters on the criterions of Danger and Distress provide the smoking gun of this rebuttal.

References

1. Hallowell, E., *Your Brain Is a Ferrari.* 2021, ADDitude, Last retrieved on November 16, 2021, from: https://www.additudemag.com/how-to-explain-adhd-to-a-child-and-build-confidence/?platform=hootsuite.
2. Chang, Z., *et al.*, *Risks and Benefits of Attention-Deficit/Hyperactivity Disorder Medication on Behavioral and Neuropsychiatric Outcomes: A Qualitative Review*

of Pharmacoepidemiology Studies Using Linked Prescription Databases. Biological Psychiatry, 2019. **86**(5): p. 335–343.

3. National Institute for Health and Care Excellence, *Attention deficit hyperactivity disorder: diagnosis and management. NICE Guideline [NG87].* 2018, Last retrieved on August 20, 2021 from: https://www.nice.org.uk/guidance/NG87.
4. Katz, S., *Assessing self-maintenance: activities of daily living, mobility, and instrumental activities of daily living.* Journal of the American Geriatrics Society, 1983. **31**(12): p. 721–727.
5. APA, *Diagnostic and Statistical Manual of Mental Disorders (DSM-5®).* 2013: American Psychiatric Association.
6. Lange, K.W., *et al.*, *The history of attention deficit hyperactivity disorder.* ADHD Attention Deficit and Hyperactivity Disorders, 2010. **2**(4): p. 241–255.
7. Smith, M., *Hyperactive Around the World? The History of ADHD in Global Perspective.* Social History of Medicine, 2017. **30**(4): p. 767–787.
8. Still, G.F., *Some abnormal psychical conditions in children.* Lancet, 1902: p. 1008–1012.
9. Barkley, R.A. and M. Fischer, *The Milwaukee Longitudinal Study of Hyperactive (ADHD) Children,* in *Attention Deficit Hyperactivity Disorder: Adult Outcome and Its Predictors.* 2017, Oxford University Press. p. 63–104.
10. APA, *Diagnostic and Statistical Manual of Mental Disorders (DSM-IV).* 1994: American Psychiatric Association.
11. Matte, B., *et al.*, *ADHD in DSM-5: a field trial in a large, representative sample of 18-to 19-year-old adults.* Psychological Medicine, 2015. **45**(2): p. 361–373.
12. Arildskov, T.W., *et al.*, *How much impairment is required for ADHD? No evidence of a discrete threshold.* Journal of Child Psychology and Psychiatry, 2021.
13. Anastopoulos, A.D., *et al.*, *Impact of child and informant gender on parent and teacher ratings of attention-deficit/hyperactivity disorder.* Psychological Assessment, 2018. **30**(10): p. 1390.
14. Cho, S.-C., *et al.*, *Are Teacher Ratings and Parent Ratings Differently Associated with Children's Intelligence and Cognitive Performance?* Psychiatry investigation, 2011. **8**(1): p. 15–21.

15. Epstein, J.N. and R.E.A. Loren, *Changes in the definition of ADHD in DSM-5: subtle but important.* Neuropsychiatry, 2013. **3**(5): p. 455.
16. Hupfeld, K.E., T.R. Abagis, and P. Shah, *Living "in the zone": hyperfocus in adult ADHD.* ADHD Attention Deficit and Hyperactivity Disorders, 2019. **11**(2): p. 191–208.
17. Groen, Y., *et al.*, *Testing the relation between ADHD and hyperfocus experiences.* Research in Developmental Disabilities, 2020. **107**: p. 103789.
18. Bioulac, S., *et al.*, *Video Game Performances Are Preserved in ADHD Children Compared With Controls.* Journal of Attention Disorders, 2012. **18**(6): p. 542–550.
19. Bavelier, D. and C.S. Green, *Enhancing Attentional Control: Lessons from Action Video Games.* Neuron, 2019. **104**(1): p. 147–163.
20. Eichenbaum, A., D. Bavelier, and C.S. Green, *Video games: Play that can do serious good.* American Journal of Play, 2014. **7**(1): p. 50–72.
21. Delisle, J. and C.M.J. Braun, *A Context for Normalizing Impulsiveness at Work for Adults with Attention Deficit/Hyperactivity Disorder (Combined Type).* Archives of Clinical Neuropsychology, 2011. **26**(7): p. 602–613.
22. Lasky, A.K., *et al.*, *ADHD in context: Young adults' reports of the impact of occupational environment on the manifestation of ADHD.* Social Science & Medicine, 2016. **161**: p. 160–168.
23. Rice, V.J., J. Butler, and D. Marra, *The relationship between symptoms of attention deficit and hyperactivity disorder and oppositional defiant disorder with soldier performance during training.* Work, 2013. **44**(Supplement 1): p. 105–114.
24. Olinover, M., *et al.*, *Strategies for improving decision making of leaders with ADHD and without ADHD in combat military context.* The Leadership Quarterly, 2021: p. 101575.
25. Verma, A. and A. Bagchi, *Attention Deficit Hyperactivity Disorder (ADHD) and Sports–What Causes ADHD and How does Sport Help deal with it?* Annals of Tropical Medicine and Public Health, 2020. **23**: p. 231–707.
26. Vlad, A.R. and A.I. Lungu, *Can a Person with Attention Deficit Hyperactivity Disorder be an Athlete?* Acta Medica Marisiensis, 2017. **63**(3).

27. Catani, M. and P. Mazzarello, *Grey Matter Leonardo da Vinci: a genius driven to distraction.* Brain, 2019. **142**(6): p. 1842–1846.

28. Archer, D., *The ADHD advantage: What you thought was a diagnosis may be your greatest strength.* 2015: Penguin.

29. Chrysikou, E.G., *Creativity in and out of (cognitive) control.* Current Opinion in Behavioral Sciences, 2019. **27**: p. 94–99.

30. White, H.A. and P. Shah, *Uninhibited imaginations: Creativity in adults with Attention-Deficit/Hyperactivity Disorder.* Personality and Individual Differences, 2006. **40**(6): p. 1121–1131.

31. Boot, N., B. Nevicka, and M. Baas, *Subclinical symptoms of attention-deficit/ hyperactivity disorder (ADHD) are associated with specific creative processes.* Personality and Individual Differences, 2017. **114**: p. 73–81.

32. Ophir, Y., *Evidence that the Diagnosis of ADHD Does Not Reflect a Chronic Bio-Medical Disease.* Ethical Human Psychology and Psychiatry, 2022. **23–2**.

33. Kooij, J.J.S., *et al., Updated European Consensus Statement on diagnosis and treatment of adult ADHD.* European Psychiatry, 2019. **56**: p. 14–34.

34. Merzon, E., *et al., ADHD as a Risk Factor for Infection With Covid-19.* Journal of Attention Disorders, 2020: p. 1087054720943271.

35. Danielson, M.L., *et al., Prevalence of Parent-Reported ADHD Diagnosis and Associated Treatment Among U.S. Children and Adolescents, 2016.* Journal of Clinical Child & Adolescent Psychology, 2018. **47**(2): p. 199–212.

36. Kessler, R.C., *et al., The World Health Organization Adult ADHD Self-Report Scale (ASRS): a short screening scale for use in the general population.* Psychological Medicine, 2005. **35**(2): p. 245–256.

37. Jensen, P.S., *et al., 3-year follow-up of the NIMH MTA study.* Journal of the American Academy of Child & Adolescent Psychiatry, 2007. **46**(8): p. 989–1002.

38. Doidge, N., *The brain that changes itself: Stories of personal triumph from the frontiers of brain science.* 2007: Penguin.

39. Rubin, B.P., *Changing brains: The emergence of the field of adult neurogenesis.* BioSocieties, 2009. **4**(4): p. 407–424.

40. Evans, W.N., M.S. Morrill, and S.T. Parente, *Measuring inappropriate medical diagnosis and treatment in survey data: The case of ADHD among school-age children.* Journal of Health Economics, 2010. **29**(5): p. 657–673.
41. Halldner, L., *et al.*, *Relative immaturity and ADHD: findings from nationwide registers, parent-and self-reports.* Journal of Child Psychology and Psychiatry, 2014. **55**(8): p. 897–904.
42. Hoshen, M.B., *et al.*, *Stimulant use for ADHD and relative age in class among children in Israel.* Pharmacoepidemiology and drug safety, 2016. **25**(6): p. 652–660.
43. Gathercole, S.E., *Cognitive approaches to the development of short-term memory.* Trends in Cognitive Sciences, 1999. **3**(11): p. 410–419.
44. Fortenbaugh, F.C., *et al.*, *Sustained Attention Across the Life Span in a Sample of 10,000: Dissociating Ability and Strategy.* Psychological Science, 2015. **26**(9): p. 1497–1510.
45. Maturo, A., *The medicalization of education: ADHD, human enhancement and academic performance.* Italian Journal of Sociology of Education, 2013. **5**(3).
46. Searight, H.R. and A.L. McLaren, *Attention-deficit hyperactivity disorder: The medicalization of misbehavior.* Journal of Clinical Psychology in Medical Settings, 1998. **5**(4): p. 467–495.
47. Armstrong, T., *The Myth of the ADHD Child, Revised Edition: 101 Ways to Improve Your Child's Behavior and Attention Span Without Drugs, Labels, or Coercion.* 2017: Penguin.
48. Stolzer, J.M., *Attention deficit hyperactivity disorder: Valid medical condition or culturally constructed myth.* Ethical Human Psychology and Psychiatry, 2009. **11**(1): p. 5–15.

“

“My brother died in a car crash because of his ADHD. My brother, Ron, had ADHD in his early childhood, and it continued all his life — which ended abruptly, six years ago, when he was 56, in a single-car accident... Ron knew what a seat belt is for. He got tickets for not wearing one. Yet his failure to use a seat belt led to his death... It is clear from many studies — some conducted by me — that irreparable harm can befall adults with ADHD when on the road. Just as clear is the fact that those with driving problems can be helped by medication. So how could the brother of an ADHD expert not receive treatment?”

Barkley, R. A. (2017). Retrieved in November, 2021 from ADDitude's website [1]

Chapter 4
Does ADHD meet the criterion of Danger?

The shuddering tragedy of Ron Barkley, the brother of Prof. Russell Barkley who leads the field of Attention Deficit Hyperactivity Disorder (ADHD) (Introduction), provokes painful questions: Could ADHD medications have saved Ron's life? Does untreated ADHD lead to premature death? I cannot imagine the grief and regret of Prof. Barkley, but I urge us to try and take some psychological distance from Ron's tragedy, and discuss the more general issue at hand: Does ADHD meet the criterion of danger for psychiatric diagnosis? And more specifically, for the millions of diagnosed children around the world who have less freedom of choice than adults whether to use ADHD medications, are they at a tangible risk for dying prematurely? Should they all use stimulant medications (that work for several hours only) on a daily basis, regardless of their school performance, to make sure that they are not in danger?

The danger criterion in psychiatric diagnosis

To answer these questions, we first need to examine the general role of the danger criterion in psychopathology. As implied in Chapter 1, the danger component is not a central, let alone, prerequisite criterion for psychiatric diagnoses. Only very few mental disorders pose an actual threat to the patients or to their surroundings. Even in the case of Major Depressive Disorder, which is a recognized risk factor for suicide behaviors, the existence of the danger component is not a required condition for making the diagnosis as the vast majority of depressed individuals will not die by suicide [2, 3]. ADHD, a much less disturbing condition that occurs mostly in childhood (Chapters 2 and 3), is no different in that regard. None of the *Diagnostic and Statistical Manual of Mental Disorders* (*DSM*) symptoms of the disorder relate to the danger component, and none of the clinicians I know require that the child will demonstrate dangerous behaviors before making the diagnosis. Nevertheless, when reviewing the literature and when reading articles on popular websites, such as the one that published Barkley's tragedy, it seems that many clinicians and researchers hold a belief that ADHD is a dangerous condition.

The consensual view about the danger criterion in ADHD

A central line of research in ADHD suggests that individuals with ADHD are somewhat *dangerous to themselves*. The hyperactivity and the poor cognitive inhibition associated with the disorder (Introduction) are believed to increase the risk of multiple dangers, including physical injuries [4], car accidents [5], sexually transmitted diseases [6], substance abuse [7], and even suicide attempts [8]. Surely enough, this long list of dangers is presumed to result in early mortality [9]. Complementing these dangers, some scholars argue that people diagnosed with ADHD are also *dangerous to others*, based on studies that found high rates of convictions and incarcerations among diagnosed individuals [10]. A Swedish study, for example, that investigated 315 prison inmates, reported that 40% of them were eligible for the diagnosis of ADHD [11] — a much higher rate than the reported prevalence of the disorder in the general population (Chapter 2).

From the alleged consensus, biomedical point of view, the multiple dangers presented above serve as a strong justification for prescribing ADHD patients with stimulant medications. In contrast to the mild and unreliable dysfunction criterion, which is evident mainly in school settings (Chapter 3), the danger component of ADHD is speculated to have severe impact on all life domains. Diagnosed individuals are therefore warned, whether explicitly or implicitly, that they put themselves at risk if they do not receive pharmacological treatment [e.g., 12]. A recent Israeli study has even argued that untreated individuals with ADHD are at a greater risk than treated individuals for being infected with the 2019 Coronavirus Disease (COVID-19) [13]. To avoid COVID-19 infections, the authors of this study (which is discussed in detail in Chapter 12), concluded that patients with ADHD should adhere to their long-term pharmacological treatment. This recommendation was given despite the lockdown and the shutdown of schools, which were applied during the first waves of the pandemic (i.e., children were not expected to be attentive and perform well in the classroom during that period). The real-life clinical picture of ADHD, however, tells a completely different story. Without underestimating the objective danger of criminal acts, or of risk behaviors, the current chapter challenges the assumption that childhood ADHD meets the criterion of danger.

The danger of premature deaths

First and foremost, let's clarify the exact risk for mortality. At first glance, conclusions from a comprehensive literature review on adverse outcomes of ADHD by Prof. Joel Nigg, a recognized expert in the field, seem unequivocal. The highlights section of the review includes a straightforward statement according to which: "ADHD is associated with elevated morbidity and mortality" [9, p. 215]. However, when reading the relevant section on early mortality within the review paper (section 5.8), the message becomes much more complex. The early mortality section in the review consists of three subsections: "Impulsivity and mortality" (section 5.8.1), "Treatment risk" (section 5.8.2), and "Suicide" (section 5.8.3). Following is a short discussion of these three risks, starting with the second risk from the stimulant medications — the popular treatment of choice for ADHD.

Treatment and mortality

The mortality risk from the medications for ADHD is, of course, not a product of the disorder itself. On the contrary, it undermines the above justification to prescribe medications for people diagnosed with ADHD, and I will come back to this troubling detail in the second part of the book (e.g., Chapter 11). Briefly, although medication-related deaths may be hard to prove and relatively rare, there is a considerable amount of evidence that stimulant medications might increase the risk for premature death, whether through cardiovascular problems [e.g., 14, 15] or through the triggering of severe mental disorders [e.g., 16] and suicide behaviors [17].

Impulsivity and mortality

The mortality risk from the impulsivity component of ADHD is described by Prof. Nigg in one paragraph only. Essentially, this paragraph relies on a single small-scale study ($N = 271$) that tracked the clinical and functional outcomes of men with and without ADHD [18]. However, even this longitudinal study, which did report of several negative outcomes of ADHD (e.g., incarcerations, mental disorders, and substance use) did **not** find statistically significant evidence for early mortality (a discussion of the non-fatal risks associated with impulsivity is provided further in this chapter).

Moreover, the researchers of this study did not consider (i.e., statistically control for) the potential, yet straightforward, artifact variables that they, themselves, measured in the study (and which therefore could not be ignored in the analyses), such as the additional mental disorder records that were collected in the study. This is a crucial methodological problem that returns in many adverse outcome studies on ADHD. Many of those additional mental disorders occur in comorbidity with ADHD (e.g., substance use disorder) and they usually serve as much stronger predictors of mortality than ADHD (see Chapter 5 for a detailed discussion of the comorbidity issue).

Finally, and alarmingly, this study did not consider the potentially dangerous effect of the very medications for ADHD, which, as discussed above, could facilitate suicide ideation and other dangerous conditions (see also in Chapter 11). These questionable methodological decisions join the authors' surprising representational decision not to mention their non-findings (contraindicative results) about premature deaths – "arguably the worst possible lifetime events" (p. 1801), as they put it – in the abstract section of their article [18]. To be fair, I wish to conclude this subsection with Prof. Nigg's own statement within the body of his article (despite his straightforward, and in my opinion, misleading, statement in the highlights section) according to which: "the life expectancy of individuals with ADHD… has not been characterized… Instead, studies addressing ADHD-related mortality issues have focused largely on the potential contributions of (a) treatment-related sudden death and (b) suicide" [9, p. 222].

ADHD and suicide

Since (a) treatment-related deaths contradict the consensual narrative regarding the danger of the disorder itself, as discussed above, we are left with (b) the risk for suicide. According to Nigg, the risk for suicide is slightly elevated in individuals with ADHD compared with the general population. This statement is based on several sources. A classic review from 2004 for example estimated that the annual suicide rate among ADHD individuals is 32–39/100,000, about three times higher than the annual suicide rate among males aged 5–24 in the US, which was estimated to be 11.2/100,000 [19]. Another national survey [20] that focused on suicide attempts (rather than on suicide completions), reported a smaller *relative risk* risk for suicide (OR = 1.5, *95% CI* = 1.1, 2.1). Importantly, both sources, as well as many others (see below), questioned the validity of the small *absolute risk* for suicide (i.e., not relative risk) that has been linked to ADHD, by admitting that the risk for suicide is much better explained by the existence of other, comorbid mental health conditions [19, 20].

A more recent systematic review of 26 articles that were published after Nigg's review, showed that, at large, the link between ADHD and suicide risk is mostly mediated through other, comorbid disorders [21]. Using structured clinical interviews, which is the gold standard data-collection methodology in psychiatric research (as they provide a comprehensive and relatively reliable information about the interviewee), the authors of this last review revealed, in a prior research, that the positive association between symptoms of ADHD and suicide risk is fully mediated by symptoms of other, comorbid disorders [22]. In fact, even believers of the dangers associated with the disorder, such as Prof. Nigg, admit that "to a substantial extent, this risk (for suicide) is mediated by co-occurring psychiatric conditions" [9, p. 223].

Chapter 5 discusses the comorbidity issue in detail but we can already conclude here that, taken together, the involvement of comorbid disorders and of pharmacological treatments for ADHD provides much more reasonable explanations for the observed (small absolute) risk of suicide, than ADHD alone. Therefore, the highlight statement, according to which: "ADHD is associated with elevated mortality" [9, p. 215] is inaccurate to say the least (for more examples of narrative misrepresentations of evidence, see Part Two and specifically Chapter 12). Instead, I propose two possibilities to understand the role of ADHD-related behaviors and treatments in suicide. In the first possibility, people with severe mental illnesses may be at a greater risk for suicide if they also tend to impulsivity (please remember that I do not deny the fact that some people are characterized with higher impulsivity than others, despite my objection to the clinical label of ADHD). In the second, and in my opinion, more disturbing possibility, individuals with ADHD-related behaviors, are prescribed with unsafe medications, which could trigger obsession, psychotic episodes, and suicide ideation (see Chapter 11). These treatment-related adverse events are especially dangerous if the child absorbs constant discouragements, insults, and humiliations in school (see Chapter 5).

The non-fatal dangers

Now, after we have established the fact that ADHD alone does not meet the rigid criterion of danger (through the lack of evidence for early mortality), we can move on to discuss some of the specific non-fatal risks and adverse outcomes, which were presented at the beginning of this chapter.

Negligent absolute risk

The discussion starts with a basic assumption in formal logic: the claim that 'the majority of A is B' is not equal to (and should not be confused with) the claim that 'the majority of B is A'. In other, more concrete words, even if the majority of prison inmates consist of individuals diagnosed with ADHD, this does not mean that most people with ADHD are likely to end up in prison. In practice, only a negligible percent of them is actually at risk for incarceration, given the high rates of ADHD (Chapter 2) and the extremely low base-rate of incarceration in the general population.

A similar, very low risk exists with regard to car accidents. Even if the *relative risk* for dangerous car accidents is increased among individuals with ADHD characteristics (a problematic assertion on its own, as discussed next), the *absolute risk* for serious accidents is still very low. Needless to say, of course, that underaged children typically do not drive cars; thus, the entire discussion regarding the increased (relative) risk for car accidents is irrelevant to ADHD children. De facto, the absolute risk for both dangers (i.e., car accidents and incarcerations) approaches zero in childhood, whether or not the child is diagnosed with ADHD.

Unfounded intimidations

Not only is the absolute risk for serious dangers negligible in childhood, there are also indications that the studies reporting of increased relative risks are sometimes biased or inaccurate (see also Chapter 12). For example, although individuals with ADHD characteristics may indeed be more adventurous — spending more time on the roads and passing the allowed driving speed — a meta-analysis examining 16 empirical studies showed that there is no evidence that ADHD individuals drive more recklessly or engage in drink driving, compared with non-ADHD drivers [23]. In fact, according to its author, this meta-analysis undermined Barkley's prior claim according to which the risk of car accidents is four times higher among drivers with ADHD compared with non-ADHD drivers [24]. Unfortunately, such unfounded intimidations are utilized by pharmaceutical companies and their representatives to depict ADHD as a dangerous condition, despite their poor validity and despite their irrelevance to children (see the previous point).

Another example of an unfounded intimidation regarding a risk that may be more relevant to children can be seen in the aforementioned study that addressed the risk for infection with COVID-19 [13]. In Chapter 12, I conduct a rigorous review of this study, but I ought to state here that the multiple distortions characterizing this study do not allow us to trust its conclusions [25]. Even if children with ADHD do have increased difficulties complying with certain COVID-19 regulations (e.g., social distancing, face masks), the study does not prove that ADHD is indeed a risk factor for COVID-19 infections, let alone that stimulant medications can reduce this risk (see Chapters 9 and 12). Moreover (for some reason), the authors did not present findings regarding severe outcomes of COVID-19 infections, such as hospitalizations, despite their accessibility to this information [25]. This danger-related information was only presented about a year later in a subsequent study from 2021 that relied on a similar and overlapping dataset [26]. This time, the study (for some reason), did not include information regarding the medications (i.e., the authors removed their previous stratification of treated and untreated cases of ADHD [27]). This strange omission leaves the reader with a bitter taste that the severe, COVID-related dangers might have been the result of the treatment, rather than the result of the disorder (see also Chapter 11). Finally, in contrast to the authors' assertion in their 2021 study regarding the increased risk for COVID-related dangers [26], evidence from the US implied that ADHD can actually be a *protective* factor against severe outcomes of COVID-19 [28]. A different research team led by Yuval Arbel, which published their findings in the same *Journal of Attention Disorders*, demonstrated evidence of an intriguing trend, in which the varying prevalence of ADHD in the US was positively linked to recovery rates from COVID-19 infections. "Rather than being a risk factor," Arbel and colleagues hypothesized, "when coping with coronavirus, ADHD also provides evolutionary advantages" [28, p. 1953].

Having said that, I am the first to admit that children with ADHD qualities, and especially those who are characterized with 'predominantly hyperactive presentation', are probably more vulnerable to various risks, such as falls, fights, and injuries (see also the discussion on neurodiversity further in this chapter). Recent studies, for example, indicated that children and adolescents with ADHD have increased risk for concussions [29, 30]. I therefore, strongly recommend parents to provide ADHD-type children with close supervision and guidance (my own children are already tired of hearing me repeat the mantra: "Mind the cars"). Yet, real and present danger is not part of the clinical picture of ADHD in childhood [31]. Even in the case of concussions, the research team of the previously cited studies conclude, in their recent literature review on this topic, that ADHD has not been proven to be associated with worse clinical outcomes or prolonged concussion recovery [32]. In addition, in their new study from 2021, the researchers did not find a link between concussions and levels of symptoms within diagnosed children [29] — a puzzling finding considering the diagnostic nature of the disorder, which relies on an artificial threshold of symptoms, usually within a continuous scale (for a similar disappearance of effects in continuous variables, see Chapter 6).

Of course, some children take more risks than others [33], but there is a large gap between this plain interpersonal difference and the claim that ADHD is a dangerous condition. Moreover, the argument that children with ADHD behaviors should receive pharmacological treatment during childhood (despite the short-term action of these drugs and the rare dangers during this period) to avoid dangerous behaviors in the future, lack logical and empirical foundations. As far as I can tell, the act of using medications to prevent (unfounded) future risks equates to buying a lottery ticket — it might feel good, but you won't win (see Chapter 9 for a detailed rebuttal of this future protection myth).

Unfounded causal mechanism

Finally, when discussing the validity of the risks that are associated with ADHD, one must hold in mine the principal methodological rule (which is recited by every first-year college student) that a statistical correlation is not equivalent to a causal relationship. In fact, Barkley himself noticed this basic rule in his 8-year longitudinal research on adolescents, where he found that Conduct Disorder (i.e., not ADHD) accounted for most of the observed negative outcomes of ADHD [34]. His subsequent research on young adults revealed that Conduct Disorder was also the more appropriate predictor of drug use, than ADHD (which yielded a similar prediction as the control group) [35]. Therefore, there is a huge gap between the plain correlation with incarceration for example, and the causal claim as if the disorder itself leads the person to engage in criminal activities.

To prove causal relationships, scientists are required to conduct Randomized Controlled Trials (RCTs), but these RCTs are, of course, not practical and not ethical in the case of criminal behaviors. Consider the following grotesque example for a potential confusion between correlation and causality. In one of my recent courses (about digital psychology), I taught a small class of undergraduate students (*N* = 34) in a highly prestigious college. During one of the lectures, I took the liberty to ask the students whether they were ever diagnosed with ADHD (they were not obligated to answer this question and they were promised that their answer would remain anonymous and would not harm them in any way). The results of this small inquiry shocked me: 19 students (54%) reported they had received a diagnosis of ADHD — a prevalence rate that is 10 times (!) higher than the estimated rates of the *DSM* (Chapter 2). I discuss the high rates of ADHD in wealthy academic institutions elsewhere [36], but I wish to utilize these rates here to illustrate the causality problem. Despite the strong correlational finding in my inquiry, I will never dare to speculate that having ADHD enabled my (great) students to get accepted to such a good school. I can think of several alternative explanations that might underlie this correlational finding (including the hypothesis that students from high socioeconomic status achieved the diagnosis to survive and succeed in such a competitive school). But even these more reasonable explanations require further empirical support.

Now, let's go back to prison (metaphorically, don't worry). Aside from the fact that a simple correlation between ADHD and incarceration does not tell us anything about the causal mechanism that enabled this link, consider the disproportionate rates of black populations in American jails. Multiple surveys found that black men in the US are five-to-eight times more likely to be incarcerated than white men [37, 38]. This statistical correlation, of course, does not mean that men of color have a unique gene that causes them to engage in criminal behaviors. In this troubling case, most scholars (to my knowledge) would probably agree that the explanation for the observed correlation is not genetic but sociological. Aside from built-in discrimination practices, a possible sociological explanation for this correlation may be that children of color attend disadvantaged schools with high dropout rates. As a result, they are more likely to find themselves roaming the streets, bored, and without proper education — all problematic conditions that increase the risk that they will eventually engage in criminal behaviors [39].

A similar logic can be applied in ADHD. Energetic and/or relatively impulsive children are bound to have more difficulties to sit still and listen to (boring) lessons (Chapter 3). They feel a strong need to move around and engage in attractive stimuli, which could disrupt the entire classroom and trigger negative responses from the teachers (Chapter 5). As a result, some of them will be expelled from school and "end up on the street". In other words, it is not the "brain disorder" that led them to engage in criminal activities; it is an outcome of a tragic intersection between the child's character and the characteristics of our educational system. Together with the low base-rate and the poor validity of the dangers associated with ADHD, the lack of a convincing causal mechanism that ties the dangers directly to the assumed neurology of ADHD, undermines the notion that ADHD meets the danger condition of psychiatric diagnosis.

Gender differences and normative neurodiversity

If we were to apply the poor logic of the prison-rates studies from above, do you know who else would be significantly more likely to end up in prison? All men would! In the US for example, men are four-to-six times more likely to be incarcerated than women [40, 41]. Yet, despite this well-known fact, most scholars, including the proponents of the biomedical paradigm, would not argue that men, in general, suffer from a built-in mental disorder. In other words, even when clear biological differences do exist (something that is yet to be proven in ADHD), they are not enough to indicate a psychopathology. Yes, men can engage in more risk-taking behaviors than women, including excessive smoking or drinking, reckless driving, or unprotected sexual activities [42], and yes, they seem to be more easily caught in physical fights [43]. However, these gender differences should not be confused with problems or pathologies.

Unfortunately, there is a strong indication that this is exactly what is happening in ADHD. Notice that, in almost all epidemiological studies (except perhaps from the ones that already documented over 20% prevalence rates of ADHD), and regardless of race or culture, males are consistently diagnosed significantly more than females [for a recent large survey, see in 44]. The current edition of the *DSM* reports that "ADHD is more frequent in males than in females in the general population, with a ratio of approximately 2:1 in children and 1.6:1 in adults" [31, p. 63]. The CDC national surveys presented in Chapter 2 indicate an even larger ratio according to which, boys are diagnosed two-to-three times more than girls. Specifically, the highest rates of ADHD in these surveys (over 20%) were observed among young male adolescents [45, 46]. Finally, the third edition of the *DSM*, which was the first to introduce the disorder as an "Attention Deficit" (see Chapter 2), reports that "the disorder is **ten times** more common in boys than in girls" [47, p. 42, bold added by Y.O.]. Correspondingly, the vast majority of children receiving stimulant medications are boys [48, 49], with previous estimates in clinic-referred samples [50] indicating an disproportionate gender gap of 9:1. In my opinion, every honest researcher should stop at this point and ask her/himself: Why is the diagnosis consistently more prevalent among boys than among girls? Are more boys born with a brain deficit?

Although some researchers tried to offer biological explanations for these (in my opinion, rhetorical) questions [e.g., 51], a simple and parsimonious answer emerges when plain gender differences are considered. Common normative boyish behaviors seem to be pathologized today unjustifiably as attention deficits or hyperactive/impulsive behaviors [52; Ch. 5, Reason #2]. Whether gender differences originate from a biological/evolutionary source or from cultural/sociological norms, decades of gender research found that males and females differ on several traits, behaviors, and preferences. From a very young age, boys seem to prefer stereotypical boy-related toys, such as vehicles, whereas girls seem to be more attracted to girl-related toys, such as dolls [53]. This gender difference is quite large (*Cohen's d* ≥ 1.60) and consistent throughout multiple studies [54]. Correspondingly, as adults, males and females usually have different job preferences. Men seem to prefer working with things, while women prefer working with people [55]. Men typically display realistic and investigative interests, whereas women display more artistic and social interests.

Different interests and preferences may originate from intrinsic personality differences. Whereas males are usually described as more assertive and open to ideas, females are described as more pleasant and agreeable [56, 57]. A large study that analyzed data from 55 nations documented such differences in multiple countries, showing again that females are somewhat more agreeable and conscientious than males [58]. It is possible then, that these differences in personality traits would also be translated to actual (and sometimes problematic) behaviors. From as early as the age when they attend preschool, boys tend to engage in significantly more physically aggressive behaviors than girls [59], and even if their academic performance resembles the performance of their female classmates, teachers tend to rate them as having more aggressive behaviors and attention difficulties [60]. Indeed, among boys, there are some who are more aggressive than others, a quality that is typically associated with ADHD, but the main gender difference regarding this quality remains robust. Similarly, ADHD-type boys may indeed suffer more physical injuries than their non-ADHD peers as mentioned above, but the main effect of gender is still dominant. A study on 6,926 adolescent athletes for example, which reported of a slightly elevated risk for concussions in ADHD among males (OR = 1.48) also found that boys, in general (20.5%), suffer more concussions than girls (14%, OR not reported) [61].

These well-researched gender differences provide a straightforward explanation for the prevalence gap in ADHD. Unfortunately, it is possible that common (i.e., not deviant), boy-related behaviors, such as physical games and risk-taking activities, are being interpreted by many teachers and parents as signs for ADHD, especially if these caregivers are females themselves. This last hypothesis has actually received support in a recent study that investigated over

1,000 teachers and 2,000 parents, who were asked to rate their students'/children's behaviors on an 18-item ADHD scale that resembles the formal diagnostic criteria of the *DSM* [62]. The results of this study showed that female teachers rated male children significantly higher on the hyperactivity subscale compared to male teachers, and that female parents rated their male children significantly higher on the inattention subscale compared with male parents. Altogether, both female parents and female teachers were more inclined, in this study, to identify boys as children at risk for ADHD than male parents and male teachers [62].

These results, in my view, should not come as a surprise to people who are familiar with the mainstream educational system in Western-oriented countries. In real-life diagnostic practices, teachers and other school personnel are usually the first to propose that the child suffers from ADHD [63]. Dr. Leonard Sax, author of the influential book "Boys Adrift" [64], has even suggested that differences in the amount of prescriptions for ADHD medications can be explained, at least partially, through the differences between teachers' perceptions and level of tolerance towards the disorder. This unique dependency on teachers' perceptions has created the exceptional medical situation discussed in Chapter 3, in which clinicians are not required, according to the current edition of the *DSM*, to observe the child's symptoms in the clinic when they make their diagnosis.

The ease with which we skip over the gender riddle (i.e., why boys are diagnosed more?), is replicated in another, related, enigma. As you might recall from the Introduction, the *DSM* delineates two clusters of symptoms (i.e., inattention and hyperactivity/impulsivity), and requires that at least six symptoms of one of these clusters be evident. Aside from the fact that these diagnostic criteria allow a wide clinical heterogeneity within one medical condition (about 16,900 different combinations of symptoms), they create a jaw-dropping phenomenon: Some of the various presentations of ADHD do not share even one identical symptom. This means that the rambunctious boy who talks a lot and runs around in the classroom shouting battle cries with his friends like a motorized jumping bean suffers from, more or less, the same brain deficit as the quiet dreamy girl who doodles beautiful looking princesses in the corner of the classroom, all by herself. Both children are presumed to have a similar executive functions problem, and, wonder of wonders, both are recommended to be treated with the same class of medications. In my opinion, this construct validity gap (Box 1, Chapter 1) should have been added directly to the ever-growing pile of validity failures (Table 4, General Discussion). However, it seems that consensus members prefer to justify this etiological puzzle through non-parsimonious stipulations. Prof. Barkley, for example, proposed a new theoretical construct called Sluggish Cognitive Tempo, which can help explain the wide heterogeneity in ADHD [65]. However, even with this new theoretical bandage, I do not see how the heterogeneous balloon, known as ADHD, can maintain its contradictory hot air (see the General Discussion).

Importantly, the heterogeneity in ADHD-related behaviors occurs also within genders. Some boys and some girls are just more active, physical, and adventurous than their peers from the same sex. This simple truth is known as neurodiversity — natural, non-pathological variations in personality and behaviors between humans [66, 67]. However, when girls demonstrate masculine type behaviors, such as the ones associated with the predominantly hyperactive/impulsive presentation of ADHD, they might encounter worse reactions and stigma from their surroundings (see also Chapter 5). Perhaps, this is why hyperactive girls are considered to be at a greater risk than boys to experience social dysfunctions and further psychiatric conditions [68, 69]. Since popular gender stereotypes dictate that girls should be polite and gentle, and perhaps play quietly with blond Barbie dolls (that have unrealistic body shapes), it is no wonder that some of these girls experience gender incongruence and shame — two risk factors of gender dysphoria and related mental disorders [70]. As long as we keep pathologizing ADHD behaviors, we doom our girls to feel incompatible. Alternatively, if we choose to perceive these behaviors as part of normal neurodiversity (see also the General Discussion), and if we dare to encourage girls to be proud of their unique (incongruent) identity, we could help them harness their 'boyish' characteristics and turn them into powerful personality strengths [71]. My beautiful and high-spirited niece who appears on the cover of this book, is a fabulous example of how parents' and teachers' positive and accepting attitude could allow adventurous and active girls to become confident and impressive heroines like Mulan (by Disney).

Essentially, the fundamental question that underlies the natural diversity existing between children is: Where does personal character end and a mental disorder begin? Like all human traits, curiosity and a taste for adventure have both advantages and disadvantages. A teenager at risk for sexually transmitted diseases is probably also a teenager that is open to exciting sexual experiences. A young adult at risk for a motorcycle accident is probably also a person who enjoys extreme sports activities, such as mountain climbing or skydiving. And yes, some of them have had multiple troubles in school as children, but this does not mean that they suffer from a neurodevelopmental disorder.

The evolutionary bright side of hyperactivity and impulsivity

The very fact that risk-taking and extreme activities are often accompanied by subjective feelings of pleasure may serve as an indication for the evolutionary value of this trait (consider, for example, the thrill of amusement and water parks). Correspondingly, people with ADHD characteristics can harness the advantages of their tendency to hyperactivity and impulsivity to lead rich and exciting lives. As adults, they might prefer challenging, high-risk occupations and become successful firemen, construction workers, or army officers [75–75]. Alternatively, they might choose to leverage their boldness and creativity and become entrepreneurs, leaders, or CEOs of high-risk high-gain start-up companies. Psychiatrist Dr. Dale Archer even hypothesized that the risk-taking tendency associated with ADHD survived throughout history because it had a distinct evolutionary advantage for our species [76].

An influential public intellectual that represents the evolutionary-psychology perspective on ADHD is Thom Hartmann. In one of his must-read books, Hartmann offered a fascinating reframing for ADHD suggesting that individuals with ADHD-like traits are not disordered but "hunters in a farmer world" [77]. Back in the historical hunter-gatherer society, Hartman theorizes, risk-taking and impulsivity were probably considered virtuous personality strengths because they allowed ADHD-type hunters to monitor food and threats (distractibility) and engage in abrupt, high-risk actions (impulsivity/ risk-taking) bravely without hesitation [77]. The fact that so many children are characterized with ADHD-like traits (Chapter 2) suggests, from this perspective, that these traits must have had an evolutionary advantage that allowed their survival.

In other words, in contrast to the alleged consensus regarding the dangerous nature of ADHD, from this evolutionary/anthropological point of view, ADHD can be seen as a context-dependent trait that contributes to the person/society survivability in certain environments (perhaps in battles or nature disasters) [78, 79]. This is because ADHD "hunters" are often prepared for action. They are capable of tracking complex and moving targets, while paying some attention to the entire environment. There are even indications from pure biogenetic research that certain genetic variations, which are associated with novelty-seeking, impulsivity, and hyperactivity, have some evolutionary advantage, in certain contexts [80, 81]. Indeed, these ADHD-like traits may be less appreciated in modern schools, but with proper guidance, matched educational and occupational environments, and especially without discouraging labels, children who possess these hunter-like qualities can grow up to be fruitful and valuable members of society [72, 78]. John Chambers, the CEO of Cisco Systems and David Neeleman, the founder of five commercial airlines, are only a few examples of such successful members [76].

Empirical support for this evolutionary psychology view emerged in a small laboratory study that applied the famous "gorilla" task among college students with and without ADHD [82]. The gorilla task is a fascinating research methodology, in which participants are instructed to monitor a video showing ball-passing between a circle of players. Typically, many participants are so caught up with the task, to the point that they miss (i.e., demonstrate an inattentional blindness to) prominent stimuli, such as a gorilla walking by [83]. Apparently, participants with ADHD were significantly more aware of the typically unattended stimuli than participants without ADHD. ADHD participants were better at detecting a gorilla figure that entered the circle of players while beating her chest, and were better at noticing another typically unattended stimulus in which one of the ball players left the scene [82]. According to the authors of this study, their results support Hartmann's hypothesis that individuals with ADHD have the attentional advantages of hunters who are able to perceive information in a simultaneous manner, from both attended and unattended channels.

This bright side of ADHD may also explain why many people with ADHD are happy and sometimes even proud about their diagnosis, in a complete contrast to most other stigmatized mental disorders (Chapter 5). "If someone told me you could be normal or you could continue to have your ADD [predominantly inattentive presentation of ADHD; Y.O.]," said David Neelman, "I would take ADD… I can distill complicated facts and come up with simple solutions. I can look out on an industry with all kinds of problems and say, how can I do this better?" [76]. Apparently, many businessmen and entrepreneurs, like Neeleman, found ways to harness the advantages associated with their ADHD, rather than suffer its alleged adverse outcomes [72].

A relatively new line of research led by Prof. Johan Wiklund ties the impulsivity and hyperactivity components of ADHD to entrepreneurship and the probability of starting a business [84, 85]. A large study of over 10,000 students from dozens of universities in the Netherlands, for example, documented a relationship between ADHD-like behaviors and entrepreneurial intentions — a relationship that was partially mediated through the tendency of the students towards risk-taking [86]. Further examination of this dataset determined that the link between ADHD-symptoms and entrepreneurship exists even when the level of the symptoms meets the diagnostic threshold required for a clinical diagnosis of ADHD [87]. Specifically, the sensation-seeking, the tendency to focus on action with little premeditation, and the desire for autonomy, all seem to have a positive influence on entrepreneurship [84]. This fit between characteristics of ADHD and the business/entrepreneurship world may be explained by the entrepreneurship environment that, in some cases, appreciates speed over accuracy. Mainstream school environment in contrast, which requires children to sit still and pay sustained attention for prolonged hours to non-thrilling lessons does not seem to fit the sensation-seeking tendency of ADHD-type children. ADHD, from this perspective, can be conceptualized essentially as an "evolutionary mismatch" [78].

ADHD is not dangerous; stimulant medications are

Taken together, the evidence for real-life benefits of impulsivity and hyperactivity alongside the negligible and unreliable dangers that are associated with ADHD (see earlier in this chapter), challenge the claims that ADHD meets the criterion of danger and that it should therefore be managed constantly with stimulant medications. Not only does the treatment of choice for ADHD not protect against future adverse outcomes (see Chapter 9), it might also crush the boundless energy and spirited, sensation-seeking characteristic of ADHD-type children (Chapters 10 and 11). In clinical reality, the pharmacological treatment for ADHD is not used for prevention of dangers but for performance enhancement, mainly in academic/school settings (Chapter 3).

Unfortunately, much of the existing intimidating studies on the danger component of ADHD ignored the contributing role of sociocultural factors, as discussed earlier. In too many cases, the available studies also did not consider the disorders that might occur in comorbidity with ADHD — disorders that were repeatedly shown to be much more dangerous than ADHD. They also dismissed the inherent methodological problem in such research, in which the disorder cannot be separated from the child's sociological framework, namely the school (i.e., if a school expels restless or disruptive children, they might actually end up on the street). Finally, and most disturbingly, many studies failed to control the adverse outcomes of the pharmacological treatment of choice for ADHD, thus confusing the dangers associated with the 'illness' with the dangers associated with the 'cure'. Perhaps this is why the *DSM* criteria does not include even one symptom that is related directly to the danger criterion of psychiatric diagnosis. After all, such a critical criterion, if it were to be intrinsic to the disorder, should have been listed as a diagnostic hallmark of ADHD.

References

1. Barkley, R.A., *My brother died in a car crash because of his ADHD*, in *ADDITUDE Inside the ADHD Mind.* 2017, ADDITUDE Inside the ADHD Mind. Last retrieved on November 16, 2021 from: https://www.additudemag.com/car-accidents-personal-essay-adult-adhd/.
2. Franklin, J.C., *et al.*, *Risk factors for suicidal thoughts and behaviors: a meta-analysis of 50 years of research.* Psychological Bulletin, 2017. **143**(2): p. 187.
3. Ophir, Y., *et al.*, *The Hitchhiker's Guide to Computational Linguistics in Suicide Prevention.* Clinical Psychological Science, 2021: p. 21677026211022013.
4. Ruiz-Goikoetxea, M., *et al.*, *Risk of unintentional injuries in children and adolescents with ADHD and the impact of ADHD medications: A systematic review and meta-analysis.* Neuroscience & Biobehavioral Reviews, 2018. **84**: p. 63–71.
5. Thompson, A.L., *et al.*, *Risky driving in adolescents and young adults with childhood ADHD.* Journal of Pediatric Psychology, 2007. **32**(7): p. 745–759.
6. Hosain, G.M.M., *et al.*, *Attention Deficit Hyperactivity Symptoms and Risky Sexual Behavior in Young Adult Women.* Journal of Women's Health, 2012. **21**(4): p. 463–468.
7. Chilcoat, H.D. and N. Breslau, *Pathways from ADHD to early drug use.* Journal of the American Academy of Child & Adolescent Psychiatry, 1999. **38**(11): p. 1347–1354.
8. Huang, K.-L., *et al.*, *Risk of suicide attempts in adolescents and young adults with attention-deficit hyperactivity disorder: a nationwide longitudinal study.* The British Journal of Psychiatry, 2018. **212**(4): p. 234–238.
9. Nigg, J.T., *Attention-deficit/hyperactivity disorder and adverse health outcomes.* Clinical Psychology Review, 2013. **33**(2): p. 215–228.
10. Mohr-Jensen, C., *et al.*, *Attention-Deficit/Hyperactivity Disorder in Childhood and Adolescence and the Risk of Crime in Young Adulthood in a Danish Nationwide*

Study. Journal of the American Academy of Child & Adolescent Psychiatry, 2019. **58**(4): p. 443–452.

11. Ginsberg, Y., T. Hirvikoski, and N. Lindefors, *Attention Deficit Hyperactivity Disorder (ADHD) among longer-term prison inmates is a prevalent, persistent and disabling disorder.* BMC Psychiatry, 2010. **10**: p. 112–112.
12. Boland, H., *et al.*, *A literature review and meta-analysis on the effects of ADHD medications on functional outcomes.* Journal of Psychiatric Research, 2020. **123**: p. 21–30.
13. Merzon, E., *et al.*, *ADHD as a Risk Factor for Infection With Covid-19.* Journal of Attention Disorders, 2020. **25**(13): p. 1783–1790.
14. Amour, M.D.S., *et al.*, *What is the effect of ADHD stimulant medication on heart rate and blood pressure in a community sample of children?* Canadian Journal of Public Health, 2018. **109**(3): p. 395–400.
15. Gould, M.S., *et al.*, *Sudden Death and Use of Stimulant Medications in Youths.* American Journal of Psychiatry, 2009. **166**(9): p. 992–1001.
16. Shyu, Y.-C., *et al.*, *Attention-deficit/hyperactivity disorder, methylphenidate use and the risk of developing schizophrenia spectrum disorders: A nationwide population-based study in Taiwan.* Schizophrenia Research, 2015. **168**(1): p. 161–167.
17. McCarthy, S., *et al.*, *Mortality associated with attention-deficit hyperactivity disorder (ADHD) drug treatment.* Drug Safety, 2009. **32**(11): p. 1089–1096.
18. Klein, R.G., *et al.*, *Clinical and functional outcome of childhood attention-deficit/hyperactivity disorder 33 years later.* Archives of General Psychiatry, 2012. **69**(12): p. 1295–1303.
19. James, A., F.H. Lai, and C. Dahl, *Attention deficit hyperactivity disorder and suicide: a review of possible associations.* Acta Psychiatrica Scandinavica, 2004. **110**(6): p. 408–415.
20. Agosti, V., Y. Chen, and F.R. Levin, *Does Attention Deficit Hyperactivity Disorder increase the risk of suicide attempts?* Journal of Affective Disorders, 2011. **133**(3): p. 595–599.
21. Balazs, J. and A. Kereszteny, *Attention-deficit/hyperactivity disorder and suicide: A systematic review.* World journal of psychiatry, 2017. **7**(1): p. 44–59.

22. Balazs, J., *et al.*, *Attention-deficit hyperactivity disorder and suicidality in a treatment naïve sample of children and adolescents.* Journal of affective disorders, 2014. **152**: p. 282–287.

23. Vaa, T., *ADHD and relative risk of accidents in road traffic: A meta-analysis.* Accident Analysis & Prevention, 2014. **62**: p. 415–425.

24. Barkley, R.A., *et al.*, *Driving-related risks and outcomes of attention deficit hyperactivity disorder in adolescents and young adults: a 3-to 5-year follow-up survey.* Pediatrics, 1993. **92**(2): p. 212–218.

25. Ophir, Y. and Y. Shir-Raz, *Manipulations and Spins in Attention Disorders Research: The Case of ADHD and COVID-19.* Ethical Human Psychology and Psychiatry, 2020. **22**: p. 98–113.

26. Merzon, E., *et al.*, T*he Association between ADHD and the Severity of COVID-19 Infection.* Journal of Attention Disorders, 2021. **26**(4): p. 491–501.

27. Ophir, Y. and Y. Shir-Raz, *Discrepancies in Studies on ADHD and COVID-19 Raise Concerns Regarding the Risks of Stimulant Treatments During an Active Pandemic.* Accepted Manuscript. Ethical Human Psychology and Psychiatry.

28. Arbel, Y., *et al.*, *Can Increased Recovery Rates from Coronavirus be explained by Prevalence of ADHD? An Analysis at the US Statewide Level.* Journal of Attention Disorders, 2020. **25**(14): p. 1951–1954.

29. Cook, N.E., J.E. Karr, and G.L. Iverson, *Children with ADHD Have a Greater Lifetime History of Concussion: Results from the ABCD Study.* Journal of Neurotrauma, 2021.

30. Iverson, G.L., *et al.*, *Middle school children with attention-deficit/hyperactivity disorder have a greater concussion history.* Clinical Journal of Sport Medicine, 2021. **31**(5): p. 438–441.

31. APA, *Diagnostic and Statistical Manual of Mental Disorders (DSM-5®).* 2013: American Psychiatric Association.

32. Cook, N.E., *et al.*, *Attention-deficit/hyperactivity disorder and outcome after concussion: a systematic review.* Journal of Developmental & Behavioral Pediatrics, 2020. **41**(7): p. 571–582.

33. Pollak, Y., *et al.*, *The role of parental monitoring in mediating the link between adolescent ADHD symptoms and risk-taking behavior.* Journal of Attention Disorders, 2020. **24**(8): p. 1141–1147.
34. Barkley, R.A., *et al.*, *The Adolescent Outcome of Hyperactive Children Diagnosed by Research Criteria: I. An 8-Year Prospective Follow-up Study.* Journal of the American Academy of Child & Adolescent Psychiatry, 1990. **29**(4): p. 546–557.
35. Barkley, R.A., *et al.*, *Young adult follow-up of hyperactive children: antisocial activities and drug use.* Journal of Child Psychology and Psychiatry, 2004. **45**(2): p. 195–211.
36. Ophir, Y., *Evidence that the Diagnosis of ADHD Does Not Reflect a Chronic Bio-Medical Disease.* Ethical Human Psychology and Psychiatry, 2022. **23–2**.
37. Western, B., *The prison boom and the decline of American citizenship.* Society, 2007. **44**(5): p. 30–36.
38. Nellis, A., *The color of justice: Racial and ethnic disparity in state prisons.* 2016.
39. Morgan, H., *Restorative Justice and the School-to-Prison Pipeline: A Review of Existing Literature.* Education Sciences, 2021. **11**(4).
40. Glaze, L., *Correctional populations in the United States,* 2011, U.S. Department of Justice, Office of Justice Programs, Bureau of Justice Statistics p. 10.
41. Glaze, L. and D. Kaeble, *Correctional Populations in the United States, 2013.* 2014: U.S. Department of Justice, Office of Justice Programs, Bureau of Justice Statistics p. 14.
42. Byrnes, J.P., D.C. Miller, and W.D. Schafer, *Gender differences in risk taking: A meta-analysis.* Psychological Bulletin, 1999. **125**(3): p. 367.
43. Björkqvist, K., *Gender differences in aggression.* Current Opinion in Psychology, 2018. **19**: p. 39–42.
44. Wong, A.W.W.A. and S.D. Landes, *Expanding Understanding of Racial-Ethnic Differences in ADHD Prevalence Rates among Children to Include Asians and Alaskan Natives/American Indians.* Journal of Attention Disorders, 2021: p. 10870547211027932.

45. Danielson, M.L., *et al.*, *Prevalence of Parent-Reported ADHD Diagnosis and Associated Treatment Among U.S. Children and Adolescents, 2016.* Journal of Clinical Child & Adolescent Psychology, 2018. **47**(2): p. 199–212.
46. Visser, S.N., *et al.*, *Trends in the parent-report of health care provider-diagnosed and medicated attention-deficit/hyperactivity disorder: United States, 2003–2011.* Journal of the American Academy of Child & Adolescent Psychiatry, 2014. **53**(1): p. 34–46.
47. APA, *Diagnostic and Statistical Manual of Mental Disorders — Third Edition (DSM-III).* 1980: American Psychiatric Association (APA).
48. Fogelman, Y., *et al.*, *Prevalence of and change in the prescription of methylphenidate in Israel over a 2-year period.* CNS Drugs, 2003. **17**(12): p. 915–919.
49. Qato, D.M., *et al.*, *Prescription Medication Use Among Children and Adolescents in the United States.* Pediatrics, 2018. **142**(3): p. e20181042.
50. Gaub, M. and C.L. Carlson, *Gender differences in ADHD: A meta-analysis and critical review.* Journal of the American Academy of Child & Adolescent Psychiatry, 1997. **36**(8): p. 1036–1045.
51. Gualtieri, T. and R.E. Hicks, *An immunoreactive theory of selective male affliction.* Behavioral and Brain Sciences, 1985. **8**(3): p. 427–441.
52. Armstrong, T., *The Myth of the ADHD Child, Revised Edition: 101 Ways to Improve Your Child's Behavior and Attention Span Without Drugs, Labels, or Coercion.* 2017: Penguin.
53. Todd, B.K., *et al.*, *Sex differences in children's toy preferences: A systematic review, meta-regression, and meta-analysis.* Infant and Child Development, 2018. **27**(2): p. e2064.
54. Davis, J.T.M. and M. Hines, *How Large Are Gender Differences in Toy Preferences? A Systematic Review and Meta-Analysis of Toy Preference Research.* Archives of Sexual Behavior, 2020. **49**(2): p. 373–394.
55. Su, R., J. Rounds, and P.I. Armstrong, *Men and things, women and people: a meta-analysis of sex differences in interests.* Psychological Bulletin, 2009. **135**(6): p. 859.

56. Costa Jr, P.T., A. Terracciano, and R.R. McCrae, *Gender differences in personality traits across cultures: robust and surprising findings.* Journal of Personality and Social Psychology, 2001. **81**(2): p. 322.
57. Weisberg, Y.J., C.G. DeYoung, and J.B. Hirsh, *Gender differences in personality across the ten aspects of the Big Five.* Frontiers in Psychology, 2011. **2**: p. 178.
58. Schmitt, D.P., *et al.*, *Why can't a man be more like a woman? Sex differences in Big Five personality traits across 55 cultures.* Journal of Personality and Social Psychology, 2008. **94**(1): p. 168.
59. Ostrov, J.M. and C.F. Keating, *Gender Differences in Preschool Aggression During Free Play and Structured Interactions: An Observational Study.* Social Development, 2004. **13**(2): p. 255–277.
60. Derks, E.M., J.J. Hudziak, and D.I. Boomsma, *Why more boys than girls with ADHD receive treatment: a study of Dutch twins.* Twin Research and Human Genetics, 2007. **10**(5): p. 765–770.
61. Iverson, G.L., *et al.*, *Concussion history in adolescent athletes with attention-deficit hyperactivity disorder.* Journal of Neurotrauma, 2016. **33**(23): p. 2077–2080.
62. Anastopoulos, A.D., *et al.*, *Impact of child and informant gender on parent and teacher ratings of attention-deficit/hyperactivity disorder.* Psychological Assessment, 2018. **30**(10): p. 1390.
63. Sax, L. and K.J. Kautz, *Who First Suggests the Diagnosis of Attention-Deficit/ Hyperactivity Disorder?* The Annals of Family Medicine, 2003. **1**(3): p. 171.
64. Sax, L., *Boys adrift: The five factors driving the growing epidemic of unmotivated boys and underachieving young men.* 2016: Basic Books.
65. Becker, S.P. and R.A. Barkley, *Sluggish cognitive tempo.* Oxford textbook of attention deficit hyperactivity disorder, 2018: p. 147–153.
66. Armstrong, T., *The Power of Neurodiversity: Unleashing the Advantages of Your Differently Wired Brain (published in hardcover as Neurodiversity).* 2011: Da Capo Lifelong Books.
67. McGee, M., *Neurodiversity.* Contexts, 2012. **11**(3): p. 12–13.

68. Dalsgaard, S., *et al.*, *Conduct problems, gender and adult psychiatric outcome of children with attention-deficit hyperactivity disorder.* The British Journal of Psychiatry, 2002. **181**(5): p. 416–421.
69. Young, S., *et al.*, *The adolescent outcome of hyperactive girls: self-report of psychosocial status.* Journal of Child Psychology and Psychiatry, 2005. **46**(3): p. 255–262.
70. Dhejne, C., *et al.*, *Mental health and gender dysphoria: A review of the literature.* International Review of Psychiatry, 2016. **28**(1): p. 44–57.
71. Craig, T. and J. LaCroix, *Tomboy as Protective Identity.* Journal of Lesbian Studies, 2011. **15**(4): p. 450–465.
72. Lasky, A.K., *et al.*, *ADHD in context: Young adults' reports of the impact of occupational environment on the manifestation of ADHD.* Social Science & Medicine, 2016. **161**: p. 160–168.
73. Rice, V.J., J. Butler, and D. Marra, *The relationship between symptoms of attention deficit and hyperactivity disorder and oppositional defiant disorder with soldier performance during training.* Work, 2013. **44**(Supplement 1): p. 105–114.
74. Olinover, M., *et al.*, *Strategies for improving decision making of leaders with ADHD and without ADHD in combat military context.* The Leadership Quarterly, 2021: p. 101575.
75. Montes, K.S. and J.N. Weatherly, *The relationship between personality traits and military enlistment: an exploratory study.* Military Behavioral Health, 2014. **2**(1): p. 98–104.
76. Archer, D., *The ADHD advantage: What you thought was a diagnosis may be your greatest strength.* 2015: Penguin.
77. Hartmann, T., *ADHD: A Hunter in a Farmer's World.* 2019: Simon and Schuster.
78. Swanepoel, A., *et al.*, *How evolutionary thinking can help us to understand ADHD.* BJPsych Advances, 2017. **23**(6): p. 410–418.
79. Shelley-Tremblay, J.F. and L.A. Rosen, *Attention deficit hyperactivity disorder: An evolutionary perspective.* The Journal of Genetic Psychology, 1996. **157**(4): p. 443–453.

80. Chen, C., *et al.*, *Population migration and the variation of dopamine D4 receptor (DRD4) allele frequencies around the globe.* Evolution and Human Behavior, 1999. **20**(5): p. 309–324.
81. Eisenberg, D.T.A., *et al.*, *Dopamine receptor genetic polymorphisms and body composition in undernourished pastoralists: An exploration of nutrition indices among nomadic and recently settled Ariaal men of northern Kenya.* BMC Evolutionary Biology, 2008. **8**(1): p. 1–12.
82. Grossman, E.S., *et al.*, *Beating their chests: University students with ADHD demonstrate greater attentional abilities on an inattentional blindness paradigm.* Neuropsychology, 2015. **29**(6): p. 882.
83. Simons, D.J. and C.F. Chabris, *Gorillas in our midst: Sustained inattentional blindness for dynamic events.* perception, 1999. **28**(9): p. 1059–1074.
84. Wiklund, J., *et al.*, *ADHD, impulsivity and entrepreneurship.* Journal of Business Venturing, 2017. **32**(6): p. 627–656.
85. Wiklund, J., H. Patzelt, and D. Dimov, *Entrepreneurship and psychological disorders: How ADHD can be productively harnessed.* Journal of Business Venturing Insights, 2016. **6**: p. 14–20.
86. Verheul, I., *et al.*, *ADHD-like behavior and entrepreneurial intentions.* Small Business Economics, 2015. **45**(1): p. 85–101.
87. Lerner, D.A., I. Verheul, and R. Thurik, *Entrepreneurship and attention deficit/hyperactivity disorder: a large-scale study involving the clinical condition of ADHD.* Small Business Economics, 2019. **53**(2): p. 381–392.

“

“When I first introduced my ADHD clients to Emotional Distress Syndrome, they got it. Hell, they were living it. They didn't feel confident, despite their Ph.D.s, bank balances, and successful careers. Unless you're having a breakdown or failure, it's hard to evaluate the emotional distress in your life, the havoc it's creating... The chronic, lifelong nature of ADHD-related stress can increase to become a syndrome akin to post-traumatic stress disorder.”

Ochoa, J. (2021). *ADHD & Emotional Distress Syndrome.* Retrieved in November, 2021 from: ADDitude's website [1]

Chapter 5
Does ADHD meet the criterion of Distress?

The opening quote of this chapter touches on the last, and in my view, the most pivotal, 'D' criterion of psychiatric diagnosis — the criterion of Distress. According to its author, James Ochoa from the medical review panel of *ADDitude* (see Chapter 3), as well as multiple other representatives of the consensus, individuals with Attention Deficit Hyperactivity Disorder (ADHD) are bound to exhibit profound emotional distress throughout their lives [2]. The leading narrative regarding the distress component of ADHD may be illustrated using an 'onion layers' metaphor: The primary implications of the "brain deficit" known as ADHD, located at the heart of this medical onion, are symptoms of inattention, hyperactivity, and impulsivity (Introduction). Then, throughout life, children who experience these symptoms grow secondary layers of poor self-esteem and emotional distress. Starting from early childhood, ADHD-type children enter an ever-escalating negative loop. They are requested repeatedly by teachers and other caregivers to be attentive, sit still, be quiet, and inhibit their spontaneous movements — the very behaviors they struggle with. Bit by bit, they accumulate failures and discouraging feedbacks from their surroundings, which can threaten their self-esteem and trigger what Ochoa called an Emotional Distress Syndrome — "a chronic state of stress related to the struggle to live with ADHD" [1].

The onion layers of distress can be extremely bitter, leading many parents, including myself, to consider the benefits of pharmacological interventions. Even 'chill' parents, who are not worried about their children's academic performance, hate to see them experiencing feelings of inadequacy or inferiority. It is therefore important that we approach this sensitive topic with caution. Readers so far might be surprised to learn that I do not deny the general narrative that is reflected in the onion layers metaphor. Indeed, I would leave out the non-parsimonious medical terms of "brain deficit" and "Emotional Distress Syndrome", but I, too, fear that children with ADHD-like traits suffer more psychological distress than their peers. Nevertheless, it is also my position that, this very narrative should ring our scientific alarm bells because it exposes a key internal validity problem that can be summarized in the following question: Does ADHD cause significant distress all by itself, or is it possible that the distress is created mainly through a third, confounding variable[1], that is our modern, Western-oriented education system? This question is central to the debate underlying this book (Introduction) because if the latter is true, then we might want to conduct a major change in our education system rather than keep medicating our children as if they suffer from a genuine medical condition (for potential psycho-educational solutions that do not involve pharmacological treatments, see the General Discussion).

The inherent Gordian Knot of distress

Truth be told, the answer to the internal validity question may not be achieved through conventional scientific measures because of the presumed early onset of the disorder (Introduction and Chapter 2). When a child in a nursery school has a hard time sitting still at the morning meeting session with the kindergarten teacher, he/she is sometimes expelled from the meeting and instructed to sit quietly at the corner of the classroom without moving. Beyond the painful humiliation, we can only imagine what torture this punishment is for ADHD-type children, who, by the very definition of the label (whether medically justified or not), feel a strong need to move, talk, and be occupied with attractive stimuli (Introduction). Without being able to move around or to engage in attractive activities (e.g., a game, a story, social interaction), the punished children are almost forced to move (e.g., swing their chairs) and create their own attractive stimulus (e.g., make funny noises that attract their peers'

[1] The term 'confounding variable' is used here in its broader/literal context, that is: an interfering variable that raises a reasonable doubt that the independent variable (e.g., ADHD) impacts the outcome variable (e.g., emotional distress), through a different mechanism than the one proposed by the (biogenetic-oriented) organizing theory. A confounding variable threatens studies' internal validity, while the alternative terms of mediating/moderating variables fail to convey the internal validity problem and may be less appropriate here because the proposed third variable (i.e., school) has only one level (i.e., almost all children go to school).

attention), thus causing the kindergarten teacher to escalate her response. In other words, while the heart of the personality 'onion' can be mostly harmless, the repeated humiliations, reprimands, and behavioral oppressions these children exhibit on a daily basis, may gradually become firm layers of personal doubt, low self-esteem, and feelings of unworthiness.

De facto, we are presented with a complex situation in which we have no scientific way to isolate the primary implications that originate directly from the neurodevelopmental condition (regardless of specific settings) from the secondary distress, which is caused by the interaction between children's traits and school environments. Essentially, most of the empirical studies on ADHD are not investigating the pure concept of ADHD; they are investigating children who have a hard time sitting and concentrating — who are growing up in a system that demands of them these exact behaviors, to sit and focus, lesson after lesson, six days a week, 12 years in a row.

Whether you believe (like I do) that the symptoms of ADHD usually reflect normative behaviors of multiple children or whether you believe that the symptoms reflect organic neurological impairments, the act of sending these children to conventional schools (where these symptoms are constantly being regimented) is almost bound to cause them mental distress [3]. Indeed, I, too, send my energetic/dreamy children to such schools (I have very little choice in this matter), but I sometimes fear that this act is not really different from throwing fresh rolls at children who are allergic to gluten. Are modern schools, as suggested by Prof. Peter Gray, a leading expert in child development, simply a new form of coercion [3]? Do conventional schools control children's natural and normative behaviors and deprive them of their basic and healthy psychological need to play, using threats, punishments, and rewards [4, 5]? I, myself, am not sure what the most accurate answer to these questions is, but, as a child clinical psychologist, I deeply identify with the African proverb often used by my dear friend and great ADHD warrior, Roman Wyden (see the Acknowledgment section), according to which: "a child who is not embraced by the village will eventually burn it down to feel its warmth."

Not only do hyperactivity and impulsivity attract negative reactions by adult caregivers, the very mission of sitting quietly in a (sometimes boring) lesson can also be experienced as coercive and aversive. To illustrate this point, consider the wide-scope implications of the provocative series of studies, published in *Science* (probably the most prestigious academic journal in the world), on "the challenges of the disengaged mind" [6]. Adult individuals in these studies were asked to participate in a simple task — to spend 'only' 6–15 minutes by themselves, without their belongings (e.g., cell phone). This seemingly harmless and easy task was experienced by most participants as an inherently unpleasant mission. For many people, the lack of external stimulations was so aversive, to the point that they chose to give themselves an electric shock. A negative stimulation for these people was preferred to no stimulation at all. One can only wonder if this study resembles a typical boring lesson in school. Are children who have increased sensation-seeking needs (Chapter 4) more prone to exhibit distress during these lessons where they are often asked to sit still and sometimes do nothing stimulating? Moreover, one of the findings in this research suggested that the boring task was more difficult for males than females. In one of the studies, 67% of the participating men self-administered at least one electric shock during the boring task and the authors speculated that this gender-related finding is due to men's increased levels of sensation-seeking [6]. While this research does not specifically address the topic of this book, this last conclusion may also explain why boys receive significantly more ADHD diagnoses than girls (Chapter 4).

Indeed, the inherent Gordian knot between ADHD, schools, and distress described earlier challenges our ability to explore the origins of the distress component in ADHD. Nevertheless, findings from my own research described in Chapter 2 may shed some indirect light on this matter. Despite the alleged consensus, according to which ADHD should be treated daily, partially because it causes objective distress, regardless of school [2, 7, 8], diagnosed participants in my research barely used ADHD medications for non-school-related purposes [9]. Their main reason for using ADHD medications was to improve academic performance in school (55.6%) or in college/professional studies

(39.1%), and to improve behavior in school (15.5%). Medications were very rarely used for managing other aspects of life, such as emotional functioning (2%) or social functioning (3%), which are said to be affected by this neurodevelopmental deficit. The medications, as presented in Chapter 3, were also very rarely used during weekends, holidays, and COVID lockdowns, once again suggesting that the subjective distress that drives people to use these medications is limited to school-related contexts [9]. I am not claiming that these findings prove that ADHD-like traits cannot cause troubles outside of the school context. As mentioned in Chapter 3, all human weaknesses can reduce functioning, and perhaps even inflict stress. Yet, this gap between the implied, biomedical perception of the physicians prescribing the treatment of choice for ADHD and the actual medication-related practices of patients suggests that the clinical significance of the distress outside of school context is minimal.

The bright side of distractibility and associative thinking

Fortunately, our freedom of choice expands significantly when we finish school. As adults, we can search our own paths, and choose the ones that mostly fit our inner interests and abilities (perhaps this fact can explain the sharp decrease in ADHD rates during adulthood — see Chapter 3). There are numerous examples of children diagnosed with ADHD who grew up to be successful and thriving adults [10]. Although conventional adult life may still favor individuals with traditional academic skills, it seems significantly more suitable to the inherent *neurodiversity* that exists between human beings [11, 12]. Whereas school settings and academic expectations tend to ignore natural neuropsychological differences between children, adult life offers opportunities to thrive in non-academic environments, such as the business world or the media market (Chapters 3 and 4).

On the bright side of ADHD, many diagnosed children and adults are characterized with valuable personal strengths, such as curiosity and creativity [13, 14]. Their distractibility and impulsivity tendencies can take a positive form of courage, cognitive flexibility, fortitude, and resilience [15]. In his sweeping book on the advantages of ADHD, Dr. Dale Archer has even claimed that the very traits that form the diagnosis can be the precise traits that would make the ADHD-type individual exceptional [10]. From his point of view, individuals with ADHD may operate along a non-linear way of thinking, like a supercomputer, whereby they consider multiple aspects of a problem in a kind of a "lateral thinking that opens things up to big ideas, albeit in jumbled succession" [16, Ch. 7]. Their unique cognitive patterns may suit high adrenalin, multitasking missions and help them remain 'cool' in crisis situations [16, Ch. 8–9].

The most researched virtue in ADHD seems to be *creativity*. Indeed, the existing literature yielded mixed results, but even proponents of the disorder acknowledge the existence of a positive link between subclinical symptoms of ADHD and creativity and propose that the two concepts share some identical brain mechanisms [17]. It is possible then, that in some settings, the lessened cognitive control and lower inhibitions characterizing ADHD are translated as divergent thinking — a cognitive pattern that allows the person to explore multiple possibilities, produce original connections between distant concepts, and generate a flow of creative, even if not always practical, ideas [13, 18, 19]. Of course, not all ADHD-type individuals are gifted with increased creativity, but many of them are, thus suggesting an advantageous role of their divergent thinking and openness to experience — the two hallmarks of creative individuals [20].

A complementary prism through which the link between ADHD and creativity can be understood is emerging from the neuropsychology literature. Neuroscientist Prof. Richard Silberstein (see the Acknowledgment section) theorizes that the increased creativity characterizing ADHD-type individuals originates from their reduced inhibition of their *brain's default mode* — the 'resting mode' of the brain, during which the person is not engaged in a specific, cognitive demanding task [21] (for more information about this neurological conceptualization of ADHD, see Chapter 6).

A less formal conceptualization of this neuropsychological idea is expressed in "the power of a shower" [22] hypothesis: Whenever our brain is in its resting mode, such as during lengthy showers, bus drives, or sports activities, our mind is allowed to wander freely, to explore remote connections between concepts, and sometimes to produce unexpected ideas and solutions. Correspondingly, a primary characteristic of Eureka experiences (sometimes called Aha! moments) is their suddenness [23]. When people disengage from a problem and allow themselves to 'just wonder', utilizing their brain's resting-state activity, a solution or an insight might suddenly appear, allowing them to fly with their thoughts and present ideas outside of the box [24]. "*There is an art,*" fantasizes Douglas Adams, the brilliant science fiction author of the Hitchhiker's Guide to the Galaxy, "*how to throw yourself at the ground and miss. The first part is easy. All it requires is simply the ability to throw yourself forward with all your weight… Most people fail to miss the ground, and if they are really trying properly, the likelihood is that they will fail to miss it fairly hard. Clearly, it is the second part, the missing, which presents the difficulties. One problem is that you have to miss the ground accidentally*" [25]. In the previous chapters, I acknowledged that ADHD-type children may experience more failures and falls than their peers. In this chapter, I wish to raise the possibility that the brain's autopilot of these children, which tends to prefer the default resting mode of mind-wandering, can also be the very quality that "accidentally" helps them to fly and flow.

Once again, the optimistic perspective that is reflected in the above discussion on creativity and the art of flying does not mean that typical ADHD traits are all positive. During my clinical work, I have encountered many diagnosed children who also exhibited difficulties in emotion regulation, which were evident when they engaged in competitive games (i.e., some of them were pretty sore losers). However, I also noticed that most of them were capable of bouncing back quickly and 'forgetting' the frustrating situation. I therefore would not be surprised if their innate tendency towards associative thinking, curiosity, and distractibility would prove to be a protective personality factor that allows them to detach from negative experiences and failures and move forward to the next game or the next stimulus, quite easily.

The double-edged sword nature of ADHD may be understood from the prism of evolutionary psychology presented by Thom Hartmann (Chapter 4). If children with ADHD were to live in the historical hunter-gatherer society, they would probably thrive as courageous hunters with sharp senses [26]. However, nowadays, after the agricultural revolution, and especially after the industrial revolution (which also set in place the modern schooling of children), these hunter traits are less appreciated. No wonder that many hunter-like children are frustrated and even distressed. Yet even hunters can thrive in our farmer-industrial world. Historical prodigies, such as Albert Einstein and Leonardo da Vinci, are speculated to have had some forms of ADHD [27, 28], and many current successful figures were actually given the diagnosis, as mentioned in Chapters 3 and 4 (Olympic champion Simone Biles and Grammy-winning singer/actor Justin Timberlake are two additional examples).

"An expectable response to a common stressor"

I, myself, as you can probably guess, do not feel comfortable diagnosing people with ADHD, let alone historical figures such as Albert Einstein. However, I do wish to learn from Einstein's biography how talented ADHD-type children could be discouraged or insulted by their teachers and caregivers. "As a child, Einstein was slow to talk and was labeled the dopey one" [29, p. 431]. He was described as a "different" child who preferred to engage in quiet activities by himself. His tremendous curiosity, along with his rebellious nature, were not always appreciated by his schoolteachers and university professors. One of his professors believed that "he would never amount to much", and quite amazingly, none of them supported his wish to become a faculty member [29]. Perhaps this is why, despite no supporting evidence, people still attribute the wonderful fish quote to Einstein: "Everybody is a genius. But if you judge a fish by its ability to climb a tree, it will live its whole life believing that it is stupid."

I, of course, do not suggest that all curious and rebellious hunter-like children can become groundbreaking theoretical physicists like Einstein, but I do insist that we cannot continue to judge our cheerful and carefree fish-children by their school-related abilities. Not only does this judgment discount their strengths, it also thickens their shameful onion layers of poor self-esteem and continuous sense of failure, once again illustrating how the distress component of ADHD is likely to be environmental, rather than congenital.

To illustrate this last, crucial point, I wish to share with you a personal childhood experience. As a young adolescent, I attended a prestigious high school where the students' social status was largely determined by their basketball talent. Unfortunately for me, my genetic predispositions determined that I would be a short boy — a tricky condition for an adolescent who wishes to be popular, in such a basketball-loving school. I was consistently chosen last by my friends to be on their teams, a recurrent adverse experience that hurt my feelings and threatened my self-esteem, despite my fantastic academic performance. I did not have a genuine medical problem, but sometimes I imagine how, from a pure biomedical perspective, a *DSM*-like manual could have named my condition a Short Height Disorder (SHD). Furthering this hypothetical ironic concept, I rationalize that back then, during the 1990s, there was very limited awareness to this made-up diagnosis of SHD. It was also not acceptable to treat SHD with growth hormones or with the controversial (made-up) medical practice of 'physical stretching of short bodies'. Thus, I was unable to realize my potential and become a successful basketball player like Kobe Bryant, God rest his soul.

Although the didactic lesson from the SHD parable is relatively straightforward, please allow me to express it explicitly: We all have strengths and weaknesses. As long as our society continues to focus on the weaknesses of ADHD-type children and as long as it continues to operate measures aimed at stretching them until they fit the one-size educational uniform, these wonderful and healthy kids will continue to experience severe emotional distress. Upon reading this intuitive idea in one of my early Hebrew articles on this topic, a friend of mine, a tall and muscular ADHD businessman (and a great basketball player who had never suffered from SHD like I did), contacted me crying, with real tears that did not match his strong appearance. "This is precisely how I felt when I was child," he said honestly. My friend is still carrying with him an enormous bag of shame and pain, but the catharsis he felt when he let this insight sink in allowed him, for the first time, to tell himself that nothing was wrong with his brain and that his distressful childhood experiences were not his fault. He was a victim, like so many other adorable children, of the medical/educational consensus.

I allowed myself to bring my friend's story (after receiving his permission) because I believe that it is not anecdotal. The very criteria for ADHD do not require that the disorder include a primary outcome of distress. None of the official *DSM* symptoms specifically reflect the existence of an emotional distress and children may be joyful and lively and still be eligible for the diagnosis. I therefore suggest to return to the basic guidelines of the *DSM* and admit that the current status quo, in which the distress component mostly emerges in school-related contexts, meets the *DSM* definition of "behavior[s]... and conflicts that are primarily between the individual and [the] society" [30, p. 20]. These conflicts and behaviors fall easily under the *DSM* category of "an expectable response to a common stressor", and they should therefore be classified as "not mental disorders", in line with the explicit instructions of the psychiatric manual (p. 20).

Clinical cases that do meet the "Four Ds" criteria

But what about the small percentage of children who do suffer from pervasive distress in all, or most, life domains, regardless of their functioning at school? Some of the children diagnosed with ADHD (let's say less than 2.5% of the general population, to meet the deviance rule of thumb described in Chapter 2) are characterized with serious cognitive difficulties or extremely poor social understanding and skills, which cause people around them to perceive them as problematic and highly disturbed children [31]. A small percent of diagnosed children may also have substantial difficulties in emotion regulation — difficulties that might explain the mixing between ADHD and conduct disorders [32] and that are sometimes thought to be a core component of ADHD [33], despite their absence from the formal *DSM* criteria. Perhaps this small percentage of highly disturbed children, who meet at least two fundamental criteria of psychiatric diagnosis (e.g., deviance and serious dysfunctions or pervasive distress), in multiple life settings, do have a neuropsychiatric condition that can be called ADHD?

This question, in my opinion, is one of the most important theoretical and practical questions of this book. If a child suffers such a major distress regardless of whether it is in the context of school, if he or she is unable to perform daily tasks without help, and if he or she is having trouble maintaining reasonable social and familial relationships, then it is quite possible that this child is indeed suffering from a genuine psychopathology. Nevertheless, in these severe and rare cases, the psychiatric diagnosis should **not** be ADHD, at least not in its current formulation at the *DSM* (Figure 2). How can I be so sure? Quite simply, the aforementioned clinical manifestations of pervasive cognitive, emotional, or social problems are not part of the current *DSM* criteria for ADHD. If these severe problems were an integral part of the clinical picture of ADHD, they should have been mentioned explicitly, especially considering their impact on the child's life.

The only way to preserve the label of ADHD and use it to describe the small percent of children suffering a genuine pathology is to reconceptualize the disorder and update its diagnostic criteria. Although I call to remove this label from the *DSM* altogether, I would be the first to celebrate if the next edition of the psychiatric manual provides stricter criteria, which will include prerequisite symptoms of severe distress, pervasive dysfunctions in daily behaviors, or serious cognitive/behavior problems that extend far beyond school-related contexts. This wished-for update would prevent millions of children from being labeled falsely with a 'real' neuropsychiatric diagnosis as the vast majority of the ~10–20% of the population of children diagnosed with ADHD (Chapter 2) do not meet the pivotal criterion of severe distress or the other three criteria of psychiatric diagnosis (Figure 2). In the current situation, where we confuse normative children with children who suffer a genuine pathology, we hurt the latter. We fail to address their unique needs and we insult their parents' intelligence. This is because, in its current softened form (see also Chapter 3), ADHD is an inappropriate label to describe the severe difficulties these children experience on a daily basis.

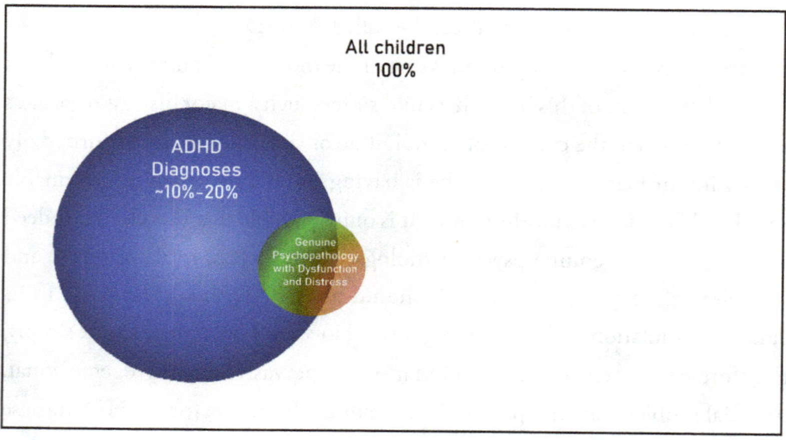

Figure 2. Illustrative Venn diagram of ADHD diagnoses and genuine (non-ADHD) psychopathology

Exceptionally poor discriminant validity

But wait a minute. If the small percent of children who **do** have psychopathology do **not** have ADHD, as suggested before, what disorder do they have? In medical discourse, this problem is part of the principal issue of *differential diagnosis* — a careful medical inspection which aims to identify the correct diagnosis, without confusing it with similar conditions. In psychiatry, for each disorder, the *DSM* typically provides a list of differential diagnosis possibilities, that is, similar conditions that should be ruled out before determining the final diagnosis. For example, the differential diagnosis section of Intellectual Disability, the neighboring disorder that shares the neurodevelopmental cluster with ADHD, comprises three potential similar conditions that should be ruled out before making the diagnosis.

The average number of differential diagnosis possibilities in this cluster of neurodevelopmental disorders (excluding ADHD) is 4.89 (SD = 1.167,

Range = 3–7). The reason I calculated these numbers is because they provide indirect estimates for the *discriminant validity* of the disorders — that is, the degree to which the phenomenology of the disorder is clearly distinct from the clinical picture of other conditions/disorders. Surprisingly, the formal list of differential diagnosis possibilities in ADHD includes **16 alternative conditions**, substantially more conditions than the average number of alternative conditions in this cluster ($t = -9.03$, $p < 0.001$). A few examples for such alternatives are: intellectual disability, anxiety disorders, depressive disorders, disruptive mood dysregulation disorder, and intermittent explosive disorder [30]. It is noted that none of the 16 alternatives constitute "normal development" or "normal variations", which are common differential diagnosis alternatives in other neurodevelopmental conditions. An even longer list of 22 differential diagnosis alternatives is offered by neurologist Richard Saul [34]. This list includes also medical (i.e., not psychiatric) conditions that might produce ADHD-like symptoms, as well as giftedness, which is of course, not a medical condition (yet).

This wealth of differential diagnosis possibilities challenges the discriminant validity of ADHD. Even proponents of the disorder agree that numerous medical and psychiatric conditions can trigger ADHD-like symptoms [35]. You know what? Forget about medical issues. Numerous life events can trigger ADHD-like symptoms. Our attention and cognitive control capabilities are easily influenced by plain factors. If the child is tired, in love, excited, or just bored, he/she would probably be less attentive. If the child is depressed, stressed out, or in conflict with his/her parents, teachers, or friends, then of course, he/she would experience attention difficulties. This means that the diagnostic mission, which should separate the pure "brain deficit" from environmental influences, and then distinguish it from a dozen alternatives, is a highly complex mission. How can clinicians differentiate, for example, between the impulsivity that characterizes ADHD and the impulsivity that characterizes intermittent explosive disorder? How can clinicians differentiate ADHD from disruptive mood dysregulation disorder if they both share similar symptoms? And most importantly, how many clinicians actually dedicate sufficient time to examine and rule out all 16 *DSM*-based differential diagnosis alternatives, not to mention the other non-psychiatric alternatives and the inconceivable options of normal development or normal variations?

The poor discriminant validity of ADHD is not only a practical clinical problem. It is a key theoretical problem of construct validity. Epidemiological research suggests that the majority of the children diagnosed with ADHD are also eligible for at least one additional diagnosis, otherwise known as a comorbid disorder [36]. The *DSM*, for example, notes that 50% of clinical cases marked as 'ADHD with combined presentation' (of both inattention and hyperactivity/impulsivity) are eligible also for a comorbid diagnosis of Oppositional Defiant Disorder (ODD). In fact, the comorbidity in ADHD is so large that Barkley himself reported that over **80%** of clinic-referred ADHD samples had at least one comorbid disorder and that over 50% of them had at least two comorbid disorders [37]. Aside from the fact that comorbidity studies typically disregard the negative artifact effects of common medications for ADHD (Chapter 4), which are known to increase the risk for comorbid psychiatric conditions (Chapters 10 and 11), such as depressive, bipolar, obsessive-compulsive, and psychotic disorders [38–42], I speculate that proponents of ADHD unintentionally formed an echo chamber of exaggerated *convergent validity*. Out of a sincere belief in the dangers posed by the disorder (Chapter 4), they created a monster — a terrifying, all-inclusive trashcan diagnosis that lost all traces of *discriminant validity* (there is typically a trade-off between these two types of *construct validity*).

De facto, this means that whenever we attribute a negative outcome to ADHD, even based on a rigorous research that makes use of a control group of healthy individuals, we cannot be sure that the negative outcome found in the experimental group (i.e., the ADHD group) is not a product of a different pathology (and when comorbid disorders are considered, they usually provide a better explanation for the observed outcome). Moreover, the all-inclusive trashcan nature of ADHD, which mixes mild/benign cases with severe cases that represent a different, and much more serious pathology (Figure 2), is bound to lead to *misinterpretation* of research results. That is because even if only a small percent of the experimental ADHD group suffers from a serious pathology, the resultant differences in adverse outcomes between the experimental and the control group would seem large and significant.

The stigma enigma

Intriguingly, many parents of ADHD children do not seem to feel comfortable with the proclaimed large comorbidity discussed beforehand. Despite the well-known connection between ADHD and ODD for example, I have encountered many parents who were not willing to accept the second psychiatric label: "Why do you say that my wonderful, energetic child has ODD?" they might challenge their doctors. "My child is perfectly healthy. It is only his ADHD that makes it difficult for him to sit still in school all day." "His ADHD", they sometimes claim, "is the only reason why he (1) often loses his temper; (2) is often angry; (3) often argues with authority figures; and (4) often refuses to comply with requests from authority figures." Although these four behaviors might indicate that the child meets the criteria for ODD [30, p. 462], many parents oppose this diagnosis, or any other psychiatric diagnosis, for that matter. It seems that ADHD has achieved a unique status in the psychiatric discourse. It is probably the only disorder in the *DSM* that maintains good public relations. The prejudice and negative stigma that are typically associated with mental disorders [43] are almost nonexistent in ADHD. In some cases, the disorder is even perceived as *egosyntonic*, that is, in harmony with the person's expectations and life goals (Chapter 1). In fact, many people brag or joke openly about having ADHD, as if it was a light handbag disorder, not like all other heavyweight psychiatric suitcases. Rather than being perceived as a heavy burden, ADHD has become a small, colorful carry-on baggage that one can bring to her/his flight of life, without paying additional charges for excess baggage.

Not everyone, of course, identifies with this last 'light baggage' metaphor, but I don't think that many people would argue that a double-digit figure of the population of children (Chapter 2) suffer significant and pervasive distress in all/most life domains. Therefore, if we wish to differentiate the tiny percent of children suffering a genuine, heavyweight pathology (that is usually also associated with negative stigma) from the rest of the children who experience light and mostly school-related difficulties (Figure 2), we should drop the Ds from the clinical label known as Attention Deficit Hyperactivity Disorder (ADHD). In most cases, ADHD is neither a brain Deficit, nor a mental Disorder. It is simply another trait or a 'mode of thought' like all other human qualities, and the secondary distress that sometimes accompanies it is not engraved in neurobiological stones. The next chapter even dares to defy these stones by challenging the consensual assumption that the primary impairments that are located at the heart of the ADHD onion originate from concrete and objective neurobiological deficits (Chapter 6).

References

1. Ochoa, J., *ADHD & Emotional Distress Syndrome*. 2021, ADDitude. Last retrieved on November 16, 2021 from: https://www.additudemag.com/adhd-emotional-overreaction-shame-blame/.
2. Kooij, J.J.S., *et al.*, *Updated European Consensus Statement on diagnosis and treatment of adult ADHD*. European Psychiatry, 2019. **56**: p. 14–34.
3. Gray, P., *The Harm of Coercive Schooling*. 2020: The Alliance for Self-Directed Education.
4. Mehta, R., D. Henriksen, and P. Mishra, *"Let Children Play!": Connecting Evolutionary Psychology and Creativity with Peter Gray*. TechTrends, 2020. **64**(5): p. 684–689.
5. Gray, P., *Free to Learn: Why Unleashing the Instinct to Play Will Make Our Children Happier*. More Self-Reliant, and Better Students for Life, 2013. **141**.
6. Wilson, T.D., *et al.*, *Just think: The challenges of the disengaged mind*. Science, 2014. **345**(6192): p. 75–77.
7. Faraone, S.V., *The scientific foundation for understanding attention-deficit/hyperactivity disorder as a valid psychiatric disorder*. European Child & Adolescent Psychiatry, 2005. **14**(1): p. 1–10.

8. Daley, D., *Attention deficit hyperactivity disorder: a review of the essential facts.* Child Care, Health and Development, 2006. **32**(2): p. 193–204.
9. Ophir, Y., *Evidence that the Diagnosis of ADHD Does Not Reflect a Chronic Bio-Medical Disease.* Ethical Human Psychology and Psychiatry, 2022. **23–2**.
10. Archer, D., *Better than normal: How what makes you different can make you exceptional.* 2012: Harmony Books.
11. Armstrong, T., *The Power of Neurodiversity: Unleashing the Advantages of Your Differently Wired Brain (published in hardcover as Neurodiversity).* 2011: Da Capo Lifelong Books.
12. McGee, M., *Neurodiversity.* Contexts, 2012. **11**(3): p. 12–13.
13. White, H.A. and P. Shah, *Uninhibited imaginations: Creativity in adults with Attention-Deficit/Hyperactivity Disorder.* Personality and Individual Differences, 2006. **40**(6): p. 1121–1131.
14. Abraham, A., *et al.*, *Creative thinking in adolescents with attention deficit hyperactivity disorder (ADHD).* Child Neuropsychology, 2006. **12**(2): p. 111–123.
15. Sedgwick, J.A., A. Merwood, and P. Asherson, *The positive aspects of attention deficit hyperactivity disorder: a qualitative investigation of successful adults with ADHD.* ADHD Attention Deficit and Hyperactivity Disorders, 2019. **11**(3): p. 241–253.
16. Archer, D., *The ADHD advantage: What you thought was a diagnosis may be your greatest strength.* 2015: Penguin.
17. Hoogman, M., *et al.*, *Creativity and ADHD: A review of behavioral studies, the effect of psychostimulants and neural underpinnings.* Neuroscience & Biobehavioral Reviews, 2020. **119**: p. 66–85.
18. Chrysikou, E.G., *Creativity in and out of (cognitive) control.* Current Opinion in Behavioral Sciences, 2019. **27**: p. 94–99.
19. Boot, N., B. Nevicka, and M. Baas, *Subclinical symptoms of attention-deficit/hyperactivity disorder (ADHD) are associated with specific creative processes.* Personality and Individual Differences, 2017. **114**: p. 73–81.
20. McCrae, R.R., *Creativity, divergent thinking, and openness to experience.* Journal of Personality and Social Psychology, 1987. **52**(6): p. 1258.

21. Silberstein, R., *et al.*, *Gender differences in parieto-frontal brain functional connectivity correlates of creativity.* Brain and Behavior, 2019. **9**(2): p. e01196.
22. Napier, N., *The Power of a Shower.* 2013, Psychology Today. Last retrieved on November 17, 2021 from: https://www.psychologytoday.com/us/blog/creativity-without-borders/201308/the-power-shower.
23. Topolinski, S. and R. Reber, *Gaining Insight Into the "Aha" Experience.* Current Directions in Psychological Science, 2010. **19**(6): p. 402–405.
24. Kounios, J., *et al.*, *The origins of insight in resting-state brain activity.* Neuropsychologia, 2008. **46**(1): p. 281–291.
25. Adams, D., *Life, the Universe and Everything: Hitchhiker's Guide to the Galaxy Book 3.* Vol. 3. 1984: Tor UK.
26. Hartmann, T., *ADHD: A Hunter in a Farmer's World.* 2019: Simon and Schuster.
27. Catani, M. and P. Mazzarello, *Grey Matter Leonardo da Vinci: a genius driven to distraction.* Brain, 2019. **142**(6): p. 1842–1846.
28. Gerber, P.J., *Employment of adults with learning disabilities and ADHD: Reasons for success and implications for resilience.* The ADHD Report, 2001. **9**(4): p. 1–5.
29. Winter Jr, F.D., *Einstein: His Life and Universe.* Baylor University Medical Center Proceedings, 2007. **20:4**: p. 431–432.
30. APA, *Diagnostic and Statistical Manual of Mental Disorders (DSM-5®).* 2013: American Psychiatric Association.
31. Coleman, W.L., *Social competence and friendship formation in adolescents with attention-deficit/hyperactivity disorder.* Adolescent Medicine: State of the Art Reviews, 2008. **19**(2): p. 278–99.
32. Kitchens, S.A., L.A. Rosén, and E.B. Braaten, *Differences in anger, aggression, depression, and anxiety between ADHD and non-ADHD children.* Journal of Attention Disorders, 1999. **3**(2): p. 77–83.
33. Barkley, R.A., *Emotional dysregulation is a core component of ADHD*, in *Attention-deficit hyperactivity disorder: A handbook for diagnosis and treatment*, R.A. Barkley, Editor. 2015, The Guilford Press. p. 81–115.
34. Saul, R., *ADHD Does not Exist: The Truth About Attention Deficit and Hyperactivity Disorder.* 2014: HarperCollins.

35. Kolar, D., *et al.*, *Treatment of adults with attention-deficit/hyperactivity disorder.* Neuropsychiatric Disease and Treatment, 2008. **4**(2): p. 389–403.
36. Walitza, S., R. Drechsler, and J. Ball, *The school child with ADHD.* Therapeutische Umschau. Revue therapeutique, 2012. **69**(8): p. 467–473.
37. Barkley, R.A. and M. Fischer, *The Milwaukee Longitudinal Study of Hyperactive (ADHD) Children.* Attention Deficit Hyperactivity Disorder: Adult Outcome and Its Predictors, 2017: p. 63.
38. Mosholder, A.D., *et al.*, *Hallucinations and other psychotic symptoms associated with the use of attention-deficit/hyperactivity disorder drugs in children.* Pediatrics, 2009. **123**(2): p. 611–616.
39. Shyu, Y.-C., *et al.*, *Attention-deficit/hyperactivity disorder, methylphenidate use and the risk of developing schizophrenia spectrum disorders: A nationwide population-based study in Taiwan.* Schizophrenia Research, 2015. **168**(1): p. 161–167.
40. Cherland, E. and R. Fitzpatrick, *Psychotic side effects of psychostimulants: a 5-year review.* The Canadian Journal of Psychiatry, 1999. **44**(8): p. 811–813.
41. Currie, J., M. Stabile, and L. Jones, *Do stimulant medications improve educational and behavioral outcomes for children with ADHD?* Journal of health economics, 2014. **37**: p. 58–69.
42. Borcherding, B.G., *et al.*, *Motor/vocal tics and compulsive behaviors on stimulant drugs: is there a common vulnerability?* Psychiatry Research, 1990. **33**(1): p. 83–94.
43. Corrigan, P.W. and A.C. Watson, *Understanding the impact of stigma on people with mental illness.* World Psychiatry, 2002. **1**(1): p. 16.

"

"ADHD was the first disorder found to be the result of a deficiency of a specific neurotransmitter — in this case, norepinephrine. ADHD brains have low levels of a neurotransmitter called norepinephrine.

Norepinephrine is linked arm-in-arm with dopamine. Dopamine is the thing that helps control the brain's reward and pleasure center. The ADHD brain has impaired activity in four functional regions of the brain. Frontal Cortex… Limbic System… Basal Ganglia… Reticular Activating System… ADHD is a complex neurological condition."

ADDitude Editors, & Silver, L. (2021). *The Neuroscience of the ADHD Brain: Truths about the ADHD brain that most people don't understand.* Last retrieved in November, 2021 from ADDitude's website [1].

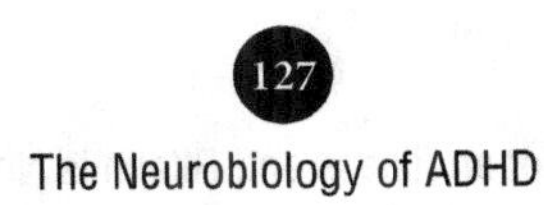

Chapter 6

Is ADHD a neurobiological deficit?

With all due respect to the "Four Ds" criteria discussed so far (Chapters 2–5), we all heard that Attention Deficit Hyperactivity Disorder (ADHD) is an objective "brain disorder" (Introduction). How can I claim that ADHD is not a valid medical illness, when "real science defines ADHD as real disorder" (Chapter 1), when the European consensus statement is so clear regarding the "neurobiological underpinnings of ADHD" [2, p. 26], and when the medical review panel of ADDitude approves the opening quotation of this chapter, which received the provocative title: "The Neuroscience of the ADHD Brain: Truths about the ADHD brain **that most people don't understand**" (bold added by Y.O.)?

Since you are reading this book, you are probably not "most people", but let's see what exactly it is that we don't understand regarding the neurobiological underpinnings of ADHD. Although the rebuttal of the scientific consensus can rely solely on the previous chapters, which exposed the numerous reliability and validity gaps in the psychiatric conceptualization of ADHD (Chapters 1–5), it is still important that we conduct an in-depth investigation of the accumulating research on the neurobiological foundations of ADHD and ask: What is the actual evidence for the deterministic biomedical position of the (alleged) consensus, as if ADHD is a chronic disorder of the brain?

Neurobiology in real-life clinical diagnosis

We shall begin our inquiry with the simple clinical truth that was presented at the beginning of the book (Chapter 1). Like all other psychopathologies, ADHD is not detected or diagnosed clinically through objective physiological measures, such as neuroimaging tools or other biological tests. The "biological revolution in psychiatry" of the previous century has not lived up to its expectations [3] and purely biological explanatory models are "woefully insufficient" when compared to actual clinical predictions, as admitted in a recent editorial article in *JAMA Psychiatry* [4]. "In the absence of clear biological markers", as stated in the *Diagnostic and Statistical Manual of Mental Disorders* (*DSM*) [5, p. 21], such simplistic biomedical perceptions have long lost their dominance in psychiatry to more complex, bio-psycho-social views [6, 7], and there are currently no indications that ADHD should be viewed differently. There are no reliable physiological measures for diagnosing ADHD, and, as discussed in the Introduction, most physicians actually believe that the diagnosis of ADHD is often given without proper medical justification [8]. If there were solid physiological tests that could signify that the person *has* the disorder, these mistakes could be easily avoided.

The clinical fact is that, like all other psychopathologies, real-life diagnoses of ADHD rely mainly on behavioral observations and subjective questionnaires. Indeed, some clinicians use more objective (non-physiological though) computer-based Continuous Performance Tests (CPTs), such as TOVA [9] or MOXO [10], which were designed to measure attention and cognitive control, but these neuropsychological tests are considered even less reliable and less valid than the more traditional diagnostic tools [11]. Specifically, the *predictive validity*, *content validity*, and *ecological validity* of these tests (Box 1, Chapter 1) are extremely poor. They produce poorer results than self-report scales and involve non-realistic tasks which do not resemble daily behaviors of children. Therefore, it is not possible to reach a conclusion about the presence or absence of ADHD based on the findings of these tests (for more information about the problematic aspects of these tests, see the 'chemical imbalance' section further in this chapter). Surprisingly, Prof. Barkley himself (Introduction) called to avoid using these tests in a recent article, which was titled: "*Neuropsychological testing is not useful in the diagnosis of ADHD: stop it (or prove it)!*" [11].

But what about the dozens of studies that documented the neurobiological foundations of ADHD? Why were their clear-cut results never translated into practical diagnostic tools in the field? What exactly can we learn from these studies regarding the validity of ADHD? Do these studies really prove that ADHD is a genuine brain deficit? The current chapter aims to provide a thorough answer to these questions, while maintaining a scientific rigor on the one hand and attempting to make the relatively complicated "truths about the ADHD brain" accessible to all readers, on the other hand.

The mind-body problem

Before entering the specific discussion regarding the neurobiological underpinnings of ADHD, we should first lay out the conventional scientific premise of the discussion, that is the way most scientists refer to the mind-body problem — the mysterious link between our physical brain and our private non-materialistic feelings, thoughts, and consciousness [12]. In contrast to the *dualism* approach, in which the mind and the body (brain) are perceived as two distinct entities (thus allowing, for example, the existence of a metaphysical soul without a physical body), the conventional scientific approach to the mind-body problem is called *monism*. In this approach, the mind and the brain are conceptualized as two dimensions of one entity, and all human experiences, even the most amorphic ones, are hypothesized to also have some physiological dimension. I am not a philosopher myself, yet I tend, like most scientists I know, to hold the latter position. Human behaviors, cognitions, and feelings, all should have physiological correlates, as far as I understand human nature. This means that our unique personality characteristics should be imprinted somehow in our brains.

Of course, no two individuals are alike, and no two have identical brains. Thus, the very existence of brain differences between people is never enough to suggest that a given person suffers from a psychiatric condition. Personality traits, such as introversion or extraversion may have neurological markers [e.g., 13, 14], yet these markers do not imply that one of these traits is a brain disorder. Another classic example is taken from gender studies. Men and women have different brains, but this fact does not imply that one of the genders (you decide which one) suffers from a psychiatric condition. Even gender identity and sexual orientation might have some neurological and genetic markers [e.g.,

15, 16]; yet these markers are by no means indicative that something is wrong with homosexual or transsexual individuals.

Homosexuality, which was officially removed from the *DSM* in 1973 [17], is actually a fundamental example of a potential confusion between plain interpersonal differences and psychiatric disorders (see the General Discussion). Today, even those who insist that the 'homosexual brain' is different from the 'heterosexual brain' acknowledge that homosexuality does not meet the Four Ds criteria of psychiatric diagnosis. The same grounding assumption should therefore be laid in the debate over the validity of ADHD. Even if the available research proves, beyond all doubt, that ADHD-like characteristics originate from specific neurobiological components (a reasonable possibility considering the conventional approach to the mind-body problem), we still need to consider the psycho-social implications of these characteristics. We should be very careful not to mix human differences (i.e., traits) with mental disorders (Chapter 1). Now, after we have established the premise of the discussion, we can move on to explore the basic question of this chapter: What does the accumulating research have to say about the neurobiological underpinnings of ADHD?

Disorder of the brain

The decades that have passed since the appearance of ADHD have yielded multiple studies that tried to track the assumed brain differences between individuals with and without ADHD [for a meta-analysis, see in: 18]. However, these studies were usually "small in size and statistical power" [19, p. 311]. It was only in 2017, when the (allegedly) solid scientific proof came along. Dozens of researchers from various places around the world conducted a mega-analysis (N = 3,242), which yielded significant volume reduction in a number of subcortical regions (mainly the amygdala, the accumbens, and the hippocampus) among participants who were diagnosed with ADHD [19]. In this mega analysis, which was published in the prestigious *Lancet Psychiatry* journal, the researchers conveyed "important messages for clinicians" in which they claimed that "patients with ADHD have altered brains" and therefore

ADHD should be conceptualized as "a disorder of the brain" [19, p. 316]. "We hope," the researchers added, that "this work will contribute to a better understanding of ADHD in the general public, and that it becomes as apparent as major depressive disorder, for example, that we label ADHD as a brain disorder" (p. 316). Surprisingly however, these dramatic statements cannot be derived from the actual findings of the mega-analysis and are not aligned with the current state of the neuroimaging literature. Following is the detailed critique.

The first (non-) finding in the mega-analysis, which challenges the notion that "patients with ADHD have altered brains", is that the volume of the examined subcortical regions did **not** differ between **adults** with and without ADHD. This disappearance of brain differences in adulthood reoccurred in a further neuroimaging investigation by the same first author, in which cortical differences in children vanished among adolescents and adults [20]. Assuming the chronic nature of ADHD, what can be the reason for this non-finding? Moreover, according to the researchers' own scientific rationale (that brain differences indicate a brain disorder), are we allowed to interpret their (non) findings regarding adults and argue that ADHD is a transient childhood illness that ends during adolescence or adulthood? Could the message for clinicians be replaced with a ground-breaking, optimistic message to parents and teachers that "the kids are alright"? According to Trudy Dehue *et al.* [21], the answer to these questions is clear: "Remarkably," they say in their response, the mega-analysis mainly teaches us that "the minor differences in children largely vanish when they grow up. This finding could have been true headline news in view of the claims by commercial pharma companies and sponsored experts that ADHD is a life-long disorder in need of life-long treatment" [21, p. 438]. Non-findings are usually not interpreted in the context of *hypothesis testing*, but in this case, not only do the non-finding regarding adults not align with the neurobiological working hypothesis about ADHD, they also corroborate with the massive evidence regarding the protective role of age in the epidemiology of the disorder (Chapter 3).

A second characteristic of the 2017 mega-analysis that challenges the explainable role of brain differences in ADHD is the fact that all the observed subcortical differences were extremely minor (*Cohen's ds* ranged from 0.1 to 0.19). In fact, in many brain regions, the confidence intervals of these differences approached zero, suggesting that the contribution of the brain differences to the explained variance in ADHD behaviors is null. Even in the brain region that showed the largest effect (*Cohen's* $d = 0.19$), the actual proportion of the explained variance (r^2) equaled 0.01. Equivalent effect sizes were observed in the 2019 study on cortical differences [20]. Indeed, many studies in the field of neuroscience are published despite their small-sized findings. However, in the case of neuroimaging studies that address a clear neurodevelopmental condition that is said to originate from a concrete biological deficit in the brain, one would expect that the findings be more substantial (i.e., that they will explain a large proportion of the variance).

A metaphor that could illustrate the negligibility of the findings in these neuroimaging analyses is an onion soup, which is made of five onions, 50 grams of butter, a cup of white wine, and many other high-quality ingredients, including four teaspoons of salt, one more teaspoon of salt than its competitor, the sweet potato soup. The argument that the observed brain differences can explain clinical differences between children with and without ADHD is equivalent to the claim that the additional smidgen of salt explains the differences in taste, texture, and particularly in the essence, between an onion soup and a sweet potato soup. Correspondingly, a recent editorial article in *JAMA Psychiatry*, the leading journal of psychiatric research and practice of the American Medical Association, concluded that small effect sizes undermine our ability to provide biological unicausal etiological explanations for psychiatric disorders and prevent us from utilizing these findings for real-life clinical diagnosis [4].

Third, the reported (negligible) effects in the 2017 mega analysis were only demonstrated when the analysis was conducted on a categorical (yes/no) variable that indicates whether the individual was diagnosed with ADHD. Strangely, the analysis of the scores of ADHD symptoms on the continuous-scale did not yield significant effects. In other words, brain volumes were not linked to symptom severity. Aside from the fact that continuous variables are usually more psychometrically informative than categorical variables, in ADHD they are also the more appropriate measures because, by definition, ADHD is a spectrum disorder. In many cases, the categorical decision whether a person has ADHD or not is extracted from a continuous scale of symptoms, based on an artificial cutoff point that was defined by humans [e.g., 22]. This means that Jonny who has four or five symptoms may not be eligible for the diagnosis, while Jessie who exhibits six symptoms could receive the diagnosis, as dictated by the *DSM* [5]. Therefore, the claim that neuroimaging measures can capture the precise, human-based, cutoff point, while missing the differences between other levels of inattention and hyperactivity/impulsivity does not make sense.

A more plausible hypothesis, in my view, is that neuroimaging tools may give us a glimpse into the neurobiology of more general cognitive tendencies (i.e., not a defined psychiatric label with specific and artificial criteria) that associate with the phenomenology of ADHD. A relatively new line of neuroimaging studies neglects the search for specific regional deficits in ADHD and focuses instead on the operational mode of larger brain networks. A leading working hypothesis, which is "unlikely to be exhaustive or equally relevant to all individuals with ADHD" [23, p. 24], postulates that (the continuous variable of) distractibility, a hallmark of ADHD, is manifested in a reduced inhibition of the *brain's default mode network* [24]. Although the precise details of the extent of the default mode network are still a matter of debate, this large network, which includes several brain regions, is activated when a person is awake but not occupied with a specific mental task. This mode, as implied in Chapter 5, can be referred to as the *resting mode* of the brain, during which the person is engaged effortlessly in daydreaming, contemplating future events or past memories, and thinking about others [25]. Using this term, we might hypothesize that individuals who tend to distractibility, shift easily to this brain default mode. This, of course, does not necessarily mean that they have a neuropsychiatric disorder (see also the discussion towards the end of this chapter).

Finally, the findings from both studies, the 2017 analysis on subcortical differences and the 2019 analysis on cortical differences [19, 20], should be interpreted in the context of the large body of research that tried to tie the disorder to observable brain differences. An early literature review of the neuroimaging studies on ADHD found that most of the studies had an incremental methodological flaw because they did not consider (i.e., statistically control for) a highly expected artifact, that is the interfering effects of the popular medications for ADHD [26]. Participants with brain differences were usually also the participants who have used medications (sometimes for lengthy periods), which impact the brain biochemistry (see Chapter 11). This review also revealed that the few studies that did separate between treated and untreated participants failed to conduct the required comparisons between these two groups, thus limiting our ability to derive conclusions regarding brain differences in ADHD. These methodological failures, as well as other biases (Chapter 12) may explain how an updated large meta-analysis of 96 neuroimaging studies showed that there is currently no significant brain regional convergences in ADHD [27]! Despite the strong statements made by proponents of the biomedical paradigm, this comprehensive and updated work challenges the *convergent validity* (Box 1) of neuroimaging findings and shows that the replication requirement — a fundamental requirement for any scientific theory — is not fulfilled in the field of brain research on ADHD. This means that, as of today, there is no clear-cut evidence for significant brain differences between individuals with and without ADHD.

Indeed, the lack of convergent validity between structural or functional neuroimaging studies is not unique to ADHD. A recent meta-analysis of multiple task-functional MRI (fMRI) measures published in *Psychological Science* (the flagship journal of the leading international Association for Psychological Science), reported evidence of a very low overall reliability, as well as poor specific types of reliability, such as test-retest reliability [28]. The authors of this meta-analysis have even concluded that these measures are "not currently suitable for brain biomarker discovery or for individual-differences research" [28, p. 792]. However, in ADHD, the reliability problem seems to extend beyond the quality of the measurements themselves. The aforementioned meta-analysis of 96 neuroimaging studies in ADHD [27] revealed that the available literature suffers from a significant risk of publication bias. This bias, which is also evident in other biomedical lines of research on ADHD (Chapter 12), produces an artificial inflation of studies that support the biomedical perception on ADHD at the expense of studies that do not align with this perception. Amazingly, despite the existence of a significant publication bias, and despite the inherent conflicts of interest that characterize the field (Chapter 12), such as the ones declared in the aforementioned studies on cortical and subcortical differences [19, 20], the existent literature fails to show an agreed upon brain deficit that associates with ADHD [27]. One can only imagine what things would have looked like if the neurobiology research were clean from biases and conflicts of interest (Chapter 12).

Chemical imbalance

Another popular notion, which was promoted during the 1990s by CHADD — the leading organization for Children and Adults with ADHD — is that the condition of ADHD results from a chemical imbalance in the brain [29]. Chemical dysregulations occur, according to supporters of the chemical imbalance theory, in key neurotransmitters such as dopamine or norepinephrine [30]. Specifically for dopamine, the ruling hypothesis is that the *reuptake process* of this neurotransmitter is amplified among children with ADHD, thus leaving insufficient levels of dopamine in the synapse — a biochemical situation that is expressed in cognitive and behavioral symptoms of ADHD [31].

To explore the validity of this hypothesis, we should first outline the general scheme of the neurotransmission process in the brain. Normally in this process, neurotransmitter molecules are (1) secreted by presynaptic neurons to the synapse, (2) stay there for a while, and (3) continue on to receptors located on postsynaptic neurons. Then, (4) in the reuptake process, the remaining neurotransmitters, which were left in the synapse, are evacuated back to the presynaptic neurons using specific proteins called transporters. This last step is speculated, as mentioned above, to be dysregulated among children with ADHD.

In a small, yet highly cited, literature review published in 2005, Thomas Spencer and colleagues documented eight studies that addressed the topic of neurotransmitter functioning in ADHD, of which six studies found high levels of dopamine transporters among ADHD children. According to the authors of this review, high levels of transporters imply that the dopamine is removed too quickly from the brain synapses, thus limiting the ability of children with ADHD to realize their full cognitive potential. 'Luckily', according to CHADD's narrative, stimulant medications can overcome this chemical imbalance through the blockage of the (presumably dysregulated) reuptake process and the retention of sufficient dopamine (and norepinephrine) levels in the synapse for a longer period of time [32]. "If treatment is successful", state the authors of a formal medication package insert (i.e., patient leaflet) — without explicitly acknowledging the chemical imbalance hypothesis — "it improves the person's **natural ability** to be attentive" (Figure 3, Chapter 10, bold added by Y.O.).

This hypothesis regarding the chemical imbalance in ADHD had received support from pioneering experiments, which used two fMRI tasks to compare the effects of stimulant medications (in these experiments, methylphenidate) on children with and without ADHD [33]. Allegedly, these experiments revealed a fascinating phenomenon. In one of the fMRI tasks (but not in the other task), the medications improved the response-inhibition performance of children with ADHD and did **not** improve it among children without ADHD (in the other task, both groups had improved). In one of the tasks, the medications also increased the striatal (basal ganglia) brain activation among ADHD children while **reducing** it among healthy children (frontal activation increased in both groups) [34]. These unexpected *selective effects* were quickly harnessed to promote a narrative according to which children with ADHD suffer from a unique brain chemical imbalance, which can be 'fixed' by adding the 'missing' pharmacological substance.

We, of course, remember from the previous section that the reliability of fMRI studies is poor [28]. However, the thrilling phenomenon of selective effects of stimulants and the studies indicating differences in neurotransmitter functioning have ignited the imagination of many. Is it possible that stimulant medications work paradoxically on ADHD children to quiet them down, while arousing (or not affecting) healthy children? Do Ritalin or Adderall only improve cognitive performance among individuals with ADHD? If you ask clinicians who are diagnosing children in their daily practice, I will not be surprised if many of them would provide a positive answer to both questions. After all, many practitioners base their clinical diagnosis on the aforementioned neuropsychological CPTs (e.g., TOVA, MOXO), which are typically administered to the child twice, before and after taking Ritalin. The validity problem of these tests aside [11], the justification of using such 'before and after' tests for diagnostic purposes is that performance improvements following the administration of stimulants is expected only among children with 'real' ADHD.

The "truth about the ADHD brain that most people don't understand" however is that the selective/paradoxical effect narrative is both logically and empirically unfounded. Although ADHD medications are perceived by many as wonder drugs, they still cannot recognize where humans drew the diagnostic line within the continuous scale of ADHD symptoms (see also the previous section on the "disorder of the brain"). There is no reason to assume that the drug works on people with six symptoms and does not work on people with four symptoms who are not eligible for the diagnosis.

De facto, stimulant medications are used today by many 'healthy' individuals as straightforward cognitive enhancers [35]. We are all familiar with the extensive non-medical use of prescribed stimulants by non-ADHD young adults who wish to enhance their academic performance [e.g., 36, 37, 38]. Indeed, some studies argue that this misuse of stimulants is essentially a type of self-treatment for those who have ADHD but were never diagnosed, but these studies only expose the ease with which false positive diagnoses can be made as well as the high abusive potential of stimulant drugs. For example, a study from George Mason University (N = 184 students aged 18–30 years) that advocated this argument found that 27.7% (!) of non-diagnosed students misused medications for ADHD, not including the 'medically justified' prescriptions given to the large percentage that were diagnosed [39]. As a side note, it is also worth mentioning that this study also reported that 27.1% of the entire sample tested positive for ADHD in the WHO Adult ADHD screening tool, thus ridiculing the deviance criterion discussed in Chapter 2 and supporting my own studies on the impossibly large rates of the disorder [40].

In addition, from an empirical point of view, there is massive evidence that the observed improvement following stimulant treatments is neither dependent on the severity of symptoms [41] nor unique to those diagnosed with this disorder [42–44]. In other words, this notion of selective or paradoxical effects of stimulants is purely a myth [45]. Stimulants work, both on individuals with ADHD and those without ADHD, and treating them as a method to diagnose ADHD in the context of neuropsychological CPTs is illogical [46].

A second "truth about the ADHD brain that most people don't understand" is that the straightforward claim about neurotransmitter dysregulations in ADHD had never received adequate support in the literature. Aside from the two studies that failed to show high levels of dopamine transporters in the aforementioned literature review from 2005 [47], four of the remaining six studies that did show evidence of elevated levels did not separate between medically treated and untreated children. This methodological shortcoming is crucial because psychostimulant use may trigger an adaptation response in which the brain produces more dopamine transporters in order to remove the externally triggered, excessive levels of dopamine in the synapse [48, see also Chapter 11]. Moreover, a study that was conducted few years later failed to replicate the findings from the 2005 review and has not demonstrated any evidence of any difference in dopamine transporter levels between individuals with and without ADHD [49]. This means that there is no clear evidence that ADHD results from a chemical imbalance in the brain — essentially like all other *DSM*-based mental disorders [e.g., 50, 51–54].

A notable remark that summarizes this section has actually been articulated recently by none other than Prof. Ronald Pies, the former editor of the consensual journal of *Psychiatric Times* and an influential psychiatrist who is not suspected to be associated with anti-psychiatry movements: "*Like the legendary Count Dracula, who could be killed only by driving a stake through his heart, some myths seem almost immortal. For more than 8 years now, I have tried to drive a stake through the heart of two myths regarding the so-called chemical imbalance theory — but with only limited success... As for the bogus chemical imbalance theory and its misattribution to the profession of psychiatry, it is time to drive the stake into its misbegotten heart*" [55, pp. 9–11]. Without entering the dispute whether psychiatry has indeed always renounced the chemical imbalance theory, this quote captures the contemporary, mainstream view regarding the popular, yet probably wrong notion that mental disorders can be traced back to specific chemical imbalances in the brain. Even consensual psychiatrists, like Pies, who believe that psychiatric labels are useful and that pharmacological interventions are required, refrain from conceptualizing psychiatric disorders as pure biochemical conditions.

Genetic differences

A final neurobiological notion is that ADHD has strong genetic foundations [2]. ADHD is conceptualized as a hereditary disorder, which has been consistently linked in the literature to specific genes [56]. In the everlasting discussion of *nature versus nurture*, ADHD falls mostly under the category of the first. The third edition of the *DSM* has even required that the symptoms of the disorder be present before the age of 3 (a criterion that was later softened, in the fourth edition to the age of 7 and in the current edition, to the age of 12), assuming that ADHD is an innate trait [57].

However, even this conventional notion has not been supported adequately. A large review of 14 years of research on molecular genetics in ADHD concludes that there is an overriding *inconsistency* in the literature on the genetic foundation of ADHD [58]. According to this review, there is currently no conclusive evidence for specific genes that could explain the appearance of ADHD behaviors. In fact, there are more studies that did *not* find genetic links to ADHD than studies that did, and the specific genes that were found (in these few studies) were not found in others. Moreover, similarly to the aforementioned literature on brain differences, the genetic literature on ADHD (mainly the first years of genetic-based research) also suffers from a significant publication bias [58]. This bias, together with the inherent conflicts of interest that characterize large portions of the biomedical literature on ADHD (Chapter 12), suggests that, not only is the current evidence regarding the biological nature of ADHD not convincing, it may also be driven by non-purely scientific considerations. The "truths about ADHD that most people don't understand" are that, like other psychopathologies, which could not be linked to specific genes [e.g., 59], we do not know which genes are involved in ADHD.

Neurobiology and diagnostic literalism

Without solid scientific grounding, reductionist neurobiological perceptions might lead to "epistemic blinders that impede progress toward valid diagnoses" [60, p. 155]. Human behaviors and experiences, as mentioned in Chapter 1, usually cannot be reduced to a small number of biological elements, and we should be very careful not to slip into *diagnostic literalism* whereby we "take mental health diagnoses for more than they are" [61, p. 2] — hypothetical abstract concepts, made up and voted by human beings [62]. Moreover, even if one day, the physical-bodily correlates of ADHD behaviors will be more pronounced and more convincing than they currently are, there is a huge gap between these hypothetical physiological markers and actual psychopathology, as described in the opening remarks of this chapter regarding the mind-body problem.

Take, for example, the novel work by Richard Silberstein (see the Acknowledgments) on brain abnormalities in ADHD [24]. Silberstein is a Professor Emeritus in cognitive neuroscience at the Swinburne University in Melbourne, Australia who promotes a relatively new line of research that focuses on brain differences in functional connectivity between ADHD and non-ADHD individuals. He also investigates brain and behavioral improvements among people diagnosed with ADHD, following the administration of stimulant medications [63]. In other words, based on his neuropsychological research, Silberstein cannot be considered as an 'ADHD denier'. Nevertheless, in his recent work on functional connectivity in creativity, he writes the following remarkable statement:

> "Our data [on brain connectivity] may also be of relevance to the issue of the relationship between ADHD and creativity [see also Chapters 3–5]... While ADHD is generally considered to comprise a set of cognitive deficits, there is growing evidence that ADHD may have had an evolutionary survival advantage, especially in hunter-gatherer societies [see also Chapter 4]... Given the... evidence that some of the genetic correlates of ADHD appear to confer survival advantages... it may be time to reconsider the current notion of ADHD as simply a cognitive deficit. Intellectual creativity is now considered one of the most important drivers of future economic well-being of nations. The fact that ADHD is associated with creativity as well offering survival advantages suggests that there may be value in **reconsidering ADHD as a particular 'mode of thought' rather than simply a 'disorder'**... This opens a wider question... has psychiatry pathologized a mode of thought, we associate with ADHD?" [64, pp. 7–8; Bold added by Y.O].

This is a good opportunity to acknowledge that Prof. Silberstein conducted a thorough scientific review of the book you are reading now (thank you so much Richard! Our correspondence and conversations were like a secret pirate treasure for me). Aside from my personal admiration of and warm gratitude to Prof. Silberstein, the reason I included his entire citation above is because it illustrates how physiological evidence is never complete without an organizing philosophical theory. Silberstein's example is quite amazing from my point of view, because it suggests that it doesn't matter if we accept the central position of this chapter that there is no convincing physiological evidence for the concrete existence of ADHD, or if we still believe that ADHD can be traced back to a definable biological source. Either way, we are obligated to rely on the philosophical assumptions that stand behind the conceptualization of any mental disorders, that is the "Four Ds" criteria of psychiatric diagnosis described in Chapter 1 [65]. Therefore, before we move on to discuss the legitimacy of the medications for ADHD (Part Two), I wish to conduct a short stopover to summarize some key conclusions from Part One regarding the validity of ADHD as a "real" neuropsychiatric disorder (see next).

References

1. ADDitude Editors and L. Silver, *The Neuroscience of the ADHD Brain: Truths about the ADHD brain that most people don't understand.* 2021, ADDitude: Inside the ADHD mind, Last retreived on November 16, 2021, from: https://www.additudemag.com/neuroscience-of-adhd-brain/.
2. Kooij, J.J.S., *et al.*, *Updated European Consensus Statement on diagnosis and treatment of adult ADHD.* European Psychiatry, 2019. **56**: p. 14–34.
3. Harrington, A., *Mind fixers: Psychiatry's troubled search for the biology of mental illness.* 2019: WW Norton & Company.
4. Paulus, M.P. and W.K. Thompson, *The Challenges and Opportunities of Small Effects: The New Normal in Academic Psychiatry.* JAMA Psychiatry, 2019. **76**(4): p. 353–354.
5. APA, *Diagnostic and Statistical Manual of Mental Disorders (DSM-5®).* 2013: American Psychiatric Association.
6. Engel, G.L., *The need for a new medical model: a challenge for biomedicine.* Science, 1977. **196**(4286): p. 129–136.
7. Lehman, B.J., D.M. David, and J.A. Gruber, *Rethinking the biopsychosocial model of health: Understanding health as a dynamic system.* Social and Personality Psychology Compass, 2017. **11**(8): p. e12328.
8. Davidovitch, M., *et al.*, *Diagnosis despite clinical ambiguity: physicians' perspectives on the rise in Autism Spectrum disorder incidence.* BMC Psychiatry, 2021. **21**(1): p. 150.
9. Leark, R.A., *et al.*, *Test of variables of attention continuous performance test.* The TOVA Company, 2007.
10. Berger, I. and G. Goldzweig, *Objective measures of attention-deficit/hyperactivity disorder: a pilot study.* IMAJ-Israel Medical Association Journal, 2010. **12**(9): p. 531.

11. Barkley, R.A., *Neuropsychological testing is not useful in the diagnosis of ADHD: Stop it (or prove it)!* The ADHD Report, 2019. **27**(2): p. 1–8.
12. Bunge, M., *The mind–body problem: A psychobiological approach.* 2014: Elsevier.
13. Nostro, A.D., *et al.*, *Predicting personality from network-based resting-state functional connectivity.* Brain Structure and Function, 2018. **223**(6): p. 2699–2719.
14. Hsu, W.-T., *et al.*, *Resting-state functional connectivity predicts neuroticism and extraversion in novel individuals.* Social Cognitive and Affective Neuroscience, 2018. **13**(2): p. 224–232.
15. Ponseti, J., *et al.*, *Homosexual women have less grey matter in perirhinal cortex than heterosexual women.* PloS one, 2007. **2**(8): p. e762.
16. Swaab, D.F., *Sexual differentiation of the human brain: relevance for gender identity, transsexualism and sexual orientation.* Gynecological Endocrinology, 2004. **19**(6): p. 301–312.
17. Drescher, J., *Out of DSM: Depathologizing Homosexuality.* Behavioral Sciences (Basel, Switzerland), 2015. **5**(4): p. 565–575.
18. Norman, L.J., *et al.*, *Structural and functional brain abnormalities in attention-deficit/hyperactivity disorder and obsessive-compulsive disorder: a comparative meta-analysis.* JAMA Psychiatry, 2016. **73**(8): p. 815–825.
19. Hoogman, M., *et al.*, *Subcortical brain volume differences in participants with attention deficit hyperactivity disorder in children and adults: a cross-sectional mega-analysis.* The Lancet Psychiatry, 2017. **4**(4): p. 310–319.
20. Hoogman, M., *et al.*, *Brain imaging of the cortex in ADHD: a coordinated analysis of large-scale clinical and population-based samples.* American Journal of Psychiatry, 2019: p. appi-ajp.
21. Dehue, T., *et al.*, *Subcortical brain volume differences in participants with attention deficit hyperactivity disorder in children and adults.* The Lancet Psychiatry, 2017. **4**(6): p. 438–439.
22. Conners, C.K., *et al.*, *The revised Conners' Parent Rating Scale (CPRS-R): factor structure, reliability, and criterion validity.* Journal of Abnormal Child Psychology, 1998. **26**(4): p. 257–268.
23. Castellanos, F.X. and E. Proal, *Large-scale brain systems in ADHD: beyond the prefrontal–striatal model.* Trends in Cognitive Sciences, 2012. **16**(1): p. 17–26.

24. Silberstein, R.B., *et al.*, *Brain functional connectivity abnormalities in attention-deficit hyperactivity disorder.* Brain and Behavior, 2016. **6**(12): p. e00583.
25. Buckner, R.L., J.R. Andrews-Hanna, and D.L. Schacter, *The brain's default network: anatomy, function, and relevance to disease.* 2008.
26. Leo, J. and D. Cohen, *Broken brains or flawed studies? A critical review of ADHD neuroimaging research.* The Journal of Mind and Behavior, 2003: p. 29–55.
27. Samea, F., *et al.*, *Brain alterations in children/adolescents with ADHD revisited: A neuroimaging meta-analysis of 96 structural and functional studies.* Neuroscience & Biobehavioral Reviews, 2019.
28. Elliott, M.L., *et al.*, *What Is the Test-Retest Reliability of Common Task-Functional MRI Measures? New Empirical Evidence and a Meta-Analysis.* Psychological Science, 2020. **31**(7): p. 792–806.
29. Whitaker, R., *Anatomy of an epidemic: Psychiatric drugs and the astonishing rise of mental illness in America.* Ethical Human Psychology and Psychiatry, 2005. 7(1): p. 23.
30. del Campo, N., *et al.*, *The roles of dopamine and noradrenaline in the pathophysiology and treatment of attention-deficit/hyperactivity disorder.* Biological Psychiatry, 2011. **69**(12): p. e145-e157.
31. Mehta, T.R., *et al.*, *Neurobiology of ADHD: A review.* Current Developmental Disorders Reports, 2019. **6**(4): p. 235–240.
32. Rosa-Neto, P., *et al.*, *Methylphenidate-evoked changes in striatal dopamine correlate with inattention and impulsivity in adolescents with attention deficit hyperactivity disorder.* NeuroImage, 2005. **25**(3): p. 868–876.
33. Vaidya, C.J. and J.D.E. Gabrieli, *Searching for a neurobiological signature of attention deficit hyperactivity disorder.* Molecular Psychiatry, 1999. **4**(3).
34. Vaidya, C.J., *et al.*, *Selective effects of methylphenidate in attention deficit hyperactivity disorder: a functional magnetic resonance study.* Proceedings of the National Academy of Sciences, 1998. **95**(24): p. 14494–14499.
35. Partridge, B.J., *et al.*, *Smart drugs "as common as coffee": media hype about neuroenhancement.* PloS one, 2011. **6**(11): p. e28416.
36. Korn, L., *et al.*, *Non-Medical Use of Prescription Stimulants for Treatment of Attention Disorders by University Students: Characteristics and Associations.* Medical Science Monitor, 2019. **25**: p. 3778.

37. DuPont, R.L., *et al.*, *Characteristics and motives of college students who engage in nonmedical use of methylphenidate.* American Journal on Addictions, 2008. **17**(3): p. 167–171.
38. Babcock, Q. and T. Byrne, *Student perceptions of methylphenidate abuse at a public liberal arts college.* Journal of American College Health, 2000. **49**(3): p. 143–145.
39. Peterkin, A.L., *et al.*, *Cognitive Performance Enhancement: Misuse or Self-Treatment?* Journal of Attention Disorders, 2010. **15**(4): p. 263–268.
40. Ophir, Y., *Evidence that the Diagnosis of ADHD Does Not Reflect a Chronic Bio-Medical Disease.* Ethical Human Psychology and Psychiatry, 2022. **23**(2).
41. Pievsky, M.A. and R.E. McGrath, *Neurocognitive effects of methylphenidate in adults with attention-deficit/hyperactivity disorder: A meta-analysis.* Neuroscience & Biobehavioral Reviews, 2018. **90**: p. 447–455.
42. Bishop, C., *et al.*, *Alerting effects of methylphenidate under basal and sleep-deprived conditions.* Experimental and Clinical Psychopharmacology, 1997. **5**(4): p. 344.
43. Roehrs, T., *et al.*, *Reinforcing and subjective effects of methylphenidate: dose and time in bed.* Experimental and Clinical Psychopharmacology, 2004. **12**(3): p. 180.
44. Volkow, N.D., *et al.*, *Evidence that methylphenidate enhances the saliency of a mathematical task by increasing dopamine in the human brain.* American Journal of Psychiatry, 2004. **161**(7): p. 1173–1180.
45. Arnsten, A.F.T., *Stimulants: therapeutic actions in ADHD.* Neuropsychopharmacology, 2006. **31**(11): p. 2376–2383.
46. Diller, L.H., *The Ritalin wars continue.* Western Journal of Medicine, 2000. **173**(6): p. 366.
47. Spencer, T.J., *et al.*, *In vivo neuroreceptor imaging in attention-deficit/hyperactivity disorder: a focus on the dopamine transporter.* Biological Psychiatry, 2005. **57**(11): p. 1293–1300.
48. Quansah, E. and T.S.C. Zetterström, *Chronic methylphenidate preferentially alters catecholamine protein targets in the parietal cortex and ventral striatum.* Neurochemistry International, 2019. **124**: p. 193–199.
49. Wang, G.-J., *et al.*, *Long-term stimulant treatment affects brain dopamine transporter level in patients with attention deficit hyperactive disorder.* PloS one, 2013. **8**(5).

50. Krishnan, V. and E.J. Nestler, *Linking Molecules to Mood: New Insight Into the Biology of Depression.* American Journal of Psychiatry, 2010. **167**(11): p. 1305–1320.
51. Jucaite, A. and S. Nyberg, *Dopaminergic hypothesis of schizophrenia: a historical perspective.* Targets and emerging therapies for schizophrenia, 2012: p. 5–35.
52. Breggin, P.R., *Rational principles of psychopharmacology for therapists, healthcare providers and clients.* Journal of Contemporary Psychotherapy, 2016. **46**(1): p. 1–13.
53. Healy, D., *Serotonin and depression.* BMJ : British Medical Journal, 2015. **350**: p. h1771.
54. Breggin, P., *The Ritalin fact book: What your doctor won't tell you about ADHD and stimulant drugs.* 2009: Da Capo Lifelong Books.
55. Pies, R.W., *Debunking the two chemical imbalance myths, again.* Psychiatric Times, 2019. **36**(8).
56. Faraone, S.V., *et al., Molecular Genetics of Attention-Deficit/Hyperactivity Disorder.* Biological Psychiatry, 2005. **57**(11): p. 1313–1323.
57. APA, *Diagnostic and Statistical Manual of Mental Disorders - Third Edition (DSM-III).* 1980: American Psychiatric Association (APA).
58. Bobb, A.J., *et al., Molecular genetic studies of ADHD: 1991 to 2004.* American Journal of Medical Genetics Part B: Neuropsychiatric Genetics, 2006. **141B**(6): p. 551–565.
59. Curtis, D., *Analysis of 50,000 exome-sequenced UK Biobank subjects fails to identify genes influencing probability of developing a mood disorder resulting in psychiatric referral.* Journal of Affective Disorders, 2021. **281**: p. 216–219.
60. Hyman, S.E., *The diagnosis of mental disorders: the problem of reification.* Annual Review of Clinical Psychology, 2010. **6**: p. 155–179.
61. Fried, E.I., *Studying mental disorders as systems, not syndromes.* PsyArXiv, 2021.
62. Kendler, K.S., *DSM disorders and their criteria: how should they inter-relate?* Psychological Medicine, 2017. **47**(12): p. 2054–2060.
63. Silberstein, R.B., *et al., Dopaminergic modulation of default mode network brain functional connectivity in attention deficit hyperactivity disorder.* Brain and Behavior, 2016. **6**(12): p. e00582.

64. Silberstein, R., *et al.*, *Gender differences in parieto-frontal brain functional connectivity correlates of creativity.* Brain and Behavior, 2019. **9**(2): p. e01196.
65. Davis, T.O., *Conceptualizing Psychiatric Disorders Using 'Four D's' of Diagnoses.* The Internet Journal of Psychiatry, 2009. **1**(1): p. 1.

Interim summary of Part One
The benefit of the doubt

As you might recall, the introductory question of this book is: Is Attention Deficit Hyperactivity Disorder (ADHD) a valid medical condition? To be more specific, this book investigates whether ADHD should be considered as the "diabetes of psychiatry", that is, a distinct and chronic neuropsychiatric condition with multiple negative implications? After laying the philosophical ground needed to answer this question (Chapter 1), Part One of this book explored the available evidence regarding the "Four Ds" criteria of psychiatric diagnosis (Chapters 2-5). The General Discussion section at the end of the book (Table 4) provides an overview of the numerous reliability and validity gaps that emerged throughout this investigation (alongside the ones that emerged in Part Two) — gaps that dismantle the theoretical concept of ADHD and undermine the justification to manage this (invalid) disorder through stimulant medications. The aim of the current Interim Summary is **not** to replace the General Discussion, but to provide readers with a short synopsis of the main rebuttal points so far (before we enter the second, and probably the more shocking part of the book that targets the medications for ADHD).

1. The rebuttal of the scientific consensus starts with the obvious. Like all other psychopathologies, real-life diagnosis of ADHD relies on behavioral observations and subjective questionnaires. To date, ADHD is not diagnosed through objective biological measures and the available biogenetic literature has very little (if any) practical diagnostic value. Therefore, in order to reject the *null hypothesis*, according to which **human beings are normal until proven otherwise**, we should first prove that the requested cluster of traits/ behaviors (i.e., the inattention, impulsivity, and hyperactivity) meets the "Four Ds" criteria of psychiatric diagnosis (or significant parts of these criteria), consisting of Deviance, Dysfunction, Danger, and Distress.

2. Amazingly, ADHD does not even meet the basic prerequisite criterion of deviance. ADHD is an extremely common condition in childhood. Its prevalence has soared dramatically within only 40 years from 3-5% to over 20% in some populations (a reliability problem on its own), and even strong believers of the disorder acknowledge today that the disorder is severely over-diagnosed. Moreover, in contrast to the assumed neurobiological etiology of the disorder, its rates are not consistent across cultures, ages, genders, and multiple other sociodemographic variables. These reliability issues cannot be explained through the consensual, biomedical view of ADHD.
3. Although the *Diagnostic and Statistical Manual of Mental Disorders* (*DSM*) list of symptoms addresses only the dysfunction criterion, its very definition is vague, subjective, and biased. Alarmingly, the dysfunction criterion has been softened in the current edition of the *DSM*, probably to fit school-related demands ("clinically significant impairment" was replaced with the terms "interfere with" and "reduce"). Children today can be eligible for the diagnosis even if they demonstrate only very little reduction in school performance, and even when they function well outside of school premises (e.g., at the clinician's office). The eligibility for ADHD, based on this criterion, also ignores the significant age differences in the prevalence of the diagnosis and the natural cognitive improvements that occur during children's development, far into their adulthood. Taken together, the current state of the diagnosis does not meet the criterion of dysfunction.
4. Childhood ADHD had also never met the criterion of danger. ADHD does not cause premature death; comorbid disorders and medications might do. Even the non-fatal dangers are rare. The absolute risk is negligible, and the relative risk is unreliable and presented in a biased manner. Unfortunately, much of the intimidating research on the 'dangerous' aspects of ADHD ignored straightforward artifact variables, such as sociocultural factors. Many of the alleged dangers of ADHD reflect plain gender differences and normative neurodiversity (boys, for example, are diagnosed two to three

times more than girls). In fact, there is a wide heterogeneity in the phenomenology of ADHD within diagnosed populations. Some presentations of the disorder do not share even one identical symptom (e.g., a loud hyperactive boy vs. a quiet dreamy girl). Moreover, boyish, risk-taking behaviors may actually have a distinct evolutionary value. Most people only use the recommended medications for ADHD (which are said to be necessary because of the assumed dangers) to enhance school-related/academic performance. The medications do not protect against future dangers and they are more likely to suppress the spirited, sensation-seeking characteristic of ADHD-type children. Perhaps this is why, despite the intimidations, the official diagnostic criteria of ADHD do not include even one symptom that is related directly to the danger criterion.

5. It is crucial to understand that the final criterion of distress cannot be separated from the child's experiences in school. Healthy children with ADHD-type behaviors are requested to behave in a way that constricts their very nature. When they fail to do so, they undergo repeated humiliations, punishments, and frustrations, which gradually become secondary layers of personal doubt, low self-esteem, and feelings of unworthiness. ADHD medications are rarely used for non-school-related purposes, suggesting that the clinical significance of the secondary distress outside of the school context is minimal. When the individual is free to choose a path that fits her/his strengths (e.g., during adulthood), the distress component of ADHD subsides, and its bright side could rise, thus suggesting, once again, that ADHD does not meet the criterion of distress.
6. The lack of the Four Ds criteria in ADHD does not mean that there are no children who suffer great distress. However, the deviant, very small percent of children suffering from clinically significant distress and/or severe dysfunction in multiple settings (i.e., not only in school) should not be confused with the large percent of (healthy) children diagnosed falsely with ADHD (Figure 2, Chapter 5). Their pervasive disabilities are not part of the current diagnostic criteria of ADHD, and it is likely that they suffer a

more serious, genuine pathology. Which pathology? The *DSM* lists 16 differential diagnosis possibilities to be considered during the clinical assessment of ADHD (significantly more possibilities than the ones provided for the rest of the neurodevelopmental conditions), thus contributing to the poor discriminant validity of the theoretical construct known as ADHD.

I am well aware that the above rebuttal points (still) reflect the view of the minority. I also acknowledge the fact that the available literature on this topic is enormous and that I might have missed important studies. Yet, one of the things that is so beautiful in scientific discourse is that "size doesn't matter", only quality, reliability, and solid methodologies do. The strength of scientific views is not measured by who wields the bigger stick or who is invited to speak at the most prestigious conference. In fact, just as in criminal law, the critical camp of any given scientific theory always has some edge over the proponents of the theory because they because they hold "the benefit of the doubt". Even if the proponent prosecutor has an army of lawyers, the critical defense needs only a reasonable doubt to undermine the allegations, because the burden of proof — the obligation to prove the theoretical crime/concept — is imposed on the party that advocates it.

In addition to the refutation arguments and the numerous validity gaps, Part One also integrated key alternative views about ADHD as formulated by influential critics, such as Sami Timimi, Thomas Armstrong, Dale Archer, and Thom Hartmann. These views add even more doubt to the mock scientific trial of ADHD, since they offer simple and straightforward alternative explanations for the emergence and maintenance of this (unfounded and unreliable) psychiatric label. Yet, it is important to remember, as mentioned in the Introduction, that these alternative views are just 'bonus' points to the main refutation. Scientifically speaking, they are not needed to the refutation of the notion that ADHD is a valid neuropsychiatric disorder, because once we stab the needles in the over-blown theoretical balloon of ADHD (H1), we ought to go back to the *null hypothesis* according to which: all children are normal unless proven otherwise (H0). We do not need to provide alternative explanations.

Perhaps you wonder, why is this refutation of the biomedical approach towards ADHD so important? Why does it matter if we label energetic/distracted children with a brain deficit or a chronic psychiatric disorder? Aside from the discouraging deterministic message in such a label, the terrifying answer to these questions pertains to the "treatment of choice" for ADHD — the highly popular stimulant medications that are prescribed to millions of diagnosed children around the world. But for the complete answer, readers should turn the page, and read the serious indictment against the efficacy, safety, and legitimacy of stimulant use presented in Part Two, that is: the comprehensive refutation of the alleged consensus regarding the medications for ADHD.

Part Two

Ritalin is Not a Cure:

A comprehensive refutation of the notion that stimulant medications are effective, safe, and morally justified

❝

"For most children, stimulant medications are a safe and effective way to relieve ADHD symptoms. As glasses help people focus their eyes to see, these medications help children with ADHD focus their thoughts better and ignore distractions. This makes them more able to pay attention and control their behavior... Studies show that about 80% of children with ADHD who are treated with stimulants improve a great deal once the right medication and dose are determined."

The American Academy of Pediatrics Parenting Website. (2019). *Common ADHD Medications & Treatments for Children.* Last retrieved on November 16, 2021 from: HealthyChildren.org [1].

Chapter 7
What is the treatment of choice for ADHD? Introducing stimulant medications

The second part of the book, as implied by the ending of the first part, consists of the main reason why I have embarked on this perilous and unrewarding voyage. The consistent increase in Attention Deficit Hyperactivity Disorder (ADHD) rates over the past decades (Chapter 2) was accompanied by a noteworthy increase in the number of children and adults using a cluster of psychoactive substances known as stimulant drugs [2–4]. Although stimulant drugs, as suggested by their name, are frequently abused for stimulating (potentially addictive) exciting sensations of high energy, euphoria, and potency, in ADHD, they are often believed to produce paradoxical calming effects (Chapter 6) and to be highly beneficial and safe. Multiple health organizations and expert consortiums determined that stimulant medications should be considered as the first-line treatment for ADHD [5–8]. These medications vary from methylphenidate (e.g., Ritalin and Concerta) to amphetamines (e.g., Adderall) and methamphetamines (e.g., Desoxyn) and their desirable effects on ADHD are achieved through their ability to increase the levels of key neurotransmitters in central parts of the brain, including in the prefrontal cortex [9] — the region of the brain that is in charge of the cognitive control functions that are said to be impaired in individuals with ADHD [10, 11].

The leading message for parents, as can be seen in the opening quotation of this chapter by the American Academy of Pediatrics, is quite simple: "As glasses help people focus their eyes to see, these medications help children with ADHD focus their thoughts better and ignore distractions" [1]. This simple (not to say simplistic) message makes sense from the point of view of the biomedical consensus. After all, children with ADHD are thought to suffer from an objective physiological condition — a tangible deficit that impacts their brain biochemistry (Introduction and Chapter 6). They, therefore, must be treated continuously with pharmacological substances; otherwise, they will not be able to manage the symptoms and risks that are bound to arise from this alleged brain deficit (remember the bicycle brakes or the diabetes metaphor from Part One). Another popular metaphor, which I myself had used in the past, to my regret (see the Prologue), is the 'broken leg' metaphor. Since the child has a vivid physiological disability that can be likened to a broken leg, the only proper solution is to provide him/her with concrete crutches — medications that will compensate for the 'chemical imbalance' in his/her brain (Chapter 6).

The simplicity of this biomedical message, which corresponds with the way most people perceive organic/physical illnesses, seems to have succeeded beyond all expectations. The CDC surveys mentioned in Chapter 2 indicated that the majority of children diagnosed with ADHD (62–69%) are using stimulant medications [12, 13]. Even very young preschool children, aged 2–5, are prescribed with these medications, despite the American Academy of Pediatrics guidelines to exclude this young group from the "first-line" recommendation and to prioritize behavior therapy over medications, at least as a first intervention [6]. Unbelievably, over 75% of medically insured children aged 2–5 in clinical care for ADHD, were given medications, according to the CDC data — a significantly higher number than those receiving other psychological services (45–54%), such as parent behavior training [14]. In fact, the medications for ADHD are so popular that they are consistently ranked at the top of the list of best-selling medications for children in the United States [15–17].

The rush for the 'magic pills' is not confined to the borders of the US only. The 'American dream' might have played a significant role in the proliferation of cognitive enhancers, such as Ritalin [18], but the alleged consensus regarding the biochemical nature of ADHD and (therefore) the favorable views about stimulant medications have spread to multiple countries around the world [19]. In Israel, for example, my beloved home, the overall prevalence of stimulant use among children has increased significantly in the past decades [20]. In my own local research (Chapter 2), I found that over 80% of diagnosed participants were prescribed with ADHD medications [21]. These rates have earned us Israelis, a silver medal in the Ritalin Olympics; this is the fourth year in a row that Israel is ranked second in the world in methylphenidate intake [22, 23]. Other leading countries are Iceland, Canada, Netherlands, and the US (see Table 2 below). Some might look at this table of mostly first world countries and ask: "Well, what's wrong with the fact that these highly advanced countries manage to provide effective and safe pharmacological treatment to so many

Table 2. Consumption rates of Methylphenidate in the 20 countries and territories reporting the highest consumption in 2019, compared with 2017 and 2018, according to the International Narcotics Control Board [23]

	S-DDD per 1,000 inhabitants per day		
Country or territory	**2017**	**2018**	**2019**
Iceland	31.94	29.05	31.77
Israel	13.95	11.75	14.84
Canada	8.09	9.49	9.19
Netherlands	7.40	7.98	8.40
United States	6.82	7.60	8.34
Spain	—	—	7.96
Denmark	7.04	7.31	7.80
Sweden	7.83	8.00	7.70
New Zealand	2.62	3.92	4.59
Switzerland	3.90	4.11	4.12
Finland	2.73	3.23	3.72
Belgium	2.36	2.86	3.10
Potugal	0.98	1.02	2.44
Germany	1.26	1.68	1.56
South Africa	1.22	1.45	1.38
Sint Maarten	0.94	1.04	1.22
Chile	1.61	1.60	1.19
Costa Rica	1.05	—	1.09
Turkey	0.00	0.96	1.01
Mexico	0.59	0.76	0.86

Note: S-DDD stands for the Defined Daily Doses for Statistical purposes.

children?" The complete answer to this seemingly innocent question is provided in Part Two of this book.

Premise, goals, and structure of Part Two

Before we begin the discussion of Part Two regarding the efficacy/safety of stimulant medications, readers who are less familiar with these drugs should know that even consensual authorities do not view these medications as harmless dietary supplements. Stimulant medications are powerful psychoactive substances, which are prohibited for use without medical prescriptions under federal drug laws. Like all psychoactive drugs, which affect the central nervous system, stimulant medications are designed to penetrate the blood-brain barrier — the specialized tissue and blood vessels that normally prevent harmful substances from reaching the brain. In that way, stimulant medications are essentially impacting the biochemical processes of our brain — that miraculous organ that makes us who we are.

In the absence of fundamental differences between stimulant medications and other psychoactive drugs, the premise of the risk-benefit discussion should be that daily usage of stimulants, even in careful medical doses, might result in physiological addiction, serious side effects, and long-term irreversible damage. If one wishes to dispel or mitigate this presumption, she/he must seriously consider the following three questions: (1) Is ADHD truly a biomedical disorder, that is, a chronic brain deficit that meets the scientific criteria of psychiatric diagnosis (and therefore requires a constant pharmacological management)? (2) Are continuous pharmacological interventions for ADHD really effective in the long term? and (3) To what extent are they harmful and dangerous?

In my view, the answer to the first question, as thoroughly discussed in Part One, is simply no. ADHD is a cluster of mostly normal behaviors found in millions of children around the world, primarily in educational frameworks. These behaviors were not proven to result from physiological deficits, and they do not meet the Four Ds criteria of psychiatric diagnosis (Part One).

Consequently, there is no scientific, let alone moral justification for "treating" these common behaviors regularly with powerful drugs that cross the blood-brain barrier. However, since many people still believe that ADHD is a valid theoretical construct, despite the numerous validity holes presented in Part One (see also Table 4 in the General Discussion), Part Two is dedicated to the remaining two questions regarding the efficacy (Chapters 8 and 9) and the safety (Chapters 10 and 11) of the first-line pharmacological treatment for ADHD. In this part, I will also describe how the medications affect the child's daily behavior (Chapter 10) and how they influence the human brain (Chapter 11). Finally, I will reflect on why most of us are unaware of the disturbing truths regarding the medications, by analyzing the biases and inherent conflicts of interests that characterize this field of research (Chapter 12).

Just before boarding, it is important to me to issue a travel advisory alert. The information about the medications presented in this part is not easy to digest. It may cause some of you to shift uncomfortably in your chair, experience unpleasant cramps, and perhaps even frustration, resistance, or anger. If, by any chance, you experience any of these sensations/feelings, please forgive me. I do not seek to instill fear or to be provocative. My sole motivation is to direct your attention — fellow scientists, clinicians, teachers, and most importantly dear parents — to massive relevant information that is being deliberately hidden from us (Chapter 12). If there is one thing that we have already learned from the COVID-19 crisis, it is the importance of receiving transparent and credible public health information. It is my belief that only when we have a credible and unbiased picture of the pharmacological treatment for ADHD, can we make the right decisions for our children.

Although 'size doesn't matter' in scientific discourse (Interim Summary of Part One), readers should know that the medication-related information brought in Part Two is based on dozens and dozens of scientific sources, including key publications by researchers who support the usage of stimulant medications in ADHD. **Part Two, of course, should not be interpreted as concrete and personal medical advice (practical medication-related decisions should be made cautiously, under proper medical supervision).**

Yet, it also cannot be dismissed as a 'conspiracy theory' from the fringe of the internet, since all the information presented in Part Two derives from well-documented literature reviews, meticulously controlled trials, longitudinal research projects, and qualitative case studies. As in the primary debate over the very conceptualization of ADHD (Introduction), the scientific consensus about stimulant medications is an illusion. Almost all the evidence against the use of stimulant medications, which is presented in the following chapters, has been published in leading and widely accepted academic journals. The evidence is usually accessible to anyone with a standard university license, but it can also be obtained directly from me, subjected to the observance of copyright laws. So, let's take a deep breath and dive into the (muddy) scientific water of the pharmacological treatment of choice for ADHD.

References

1. The American Academy of Pediatrics Parenting Website, *Common ADHD Medications & Treatments for Children*. 2019, Healthy Children.org by the American Academy of Pediatrics. Last retrieved on November 16, 2021, from: https://www.healthychildren.org/English/health-issues/conditions/adhd/Pages/Determining-ADHD-Medication-Treatments.aspx.
2. Piper, B.J., *et al.*, *Trends in use of prescription stimulants in the United States and Territories, 2006 to 2016*. PloS one, 2018. **13**(11): p. e0206100.
3. Raman, S.R., *et al.*, *Trends in attention-deficit hyperactivity disorder medication use: a retrospective observational study using population-based databases*. The Lancet Psychiatry, 2018. **5**(10): p. 824–835.
4. Burcu, M., *et al.*, *Trends in Stimulant Medication Use in Commercially Insured Youths and Adults, 2010-2014*. JAMA Psychiatry, 2016. **73**(9): p. 992–993.
5. National Institute of Mental Health, *NIH Consensus Development Conference on Diagnosis and Treatment of Attention Deficit Hyperactivity Disorder: November 16–18, 1998, William H. Natcher Conference Center, National Institutes of Health, Bethesda, Maryland*. 1998: National Institutes of Health, Continuing Medical Education.

6. American Academy of Pediatrics, *ADHD: Clinical Practice Guideline for the Diagnosis, Evaluation, and Treatment of Attention-Deficit/Hyperactivity Disorder in Children and Adolescents.* Pediatrics, 2011. **128**(5): p. 1007.
7. Bolea-Alamañac, B., *et al.*, *Evidence-based guidelines for the pharmacological management of attention deficit hyperactivity disorder: Update on recommendations from the British Association for Psychopharmacology.* Journal of Psychopharmacology, 2014. **28**(3): p. 179–203.
8. National Institute for Health and Care Excellence, *Attention deficit hyperactivity disorder: diagnosis and management. NICE Guideline [NG87].* 2018, Last retrieved on August 20, 2021 from: https://www.nice.org.uk/guidance/NG87.
9. Arnsten, A.F.T., *Stimulants: therapeutic actions in ADHD.* Neuropsychopharmacology, 2006. **31**(11): p. 2376–2383.
10. Barkley, R.A., *Behavioral inhibition, sustained attention, and executive functions: constructing a unifying theory of ADHD.* Psychological Bulletin, 1997. **121**(1): p. 65.
11. Nigg, J.T., *Is ADHD a disinhibitory disorder?* Psychological Bulletin, 2001. **127**(5): p. 571.
12. Danielson, M.L., *et al.*, *Prevalence of Parent-Reported ADHD Diagnosis and Associated Treatment Among U.S. Children and Adolescents, 2016.* Journal of Clinical Child & Adolescent Psychology, 2018. **47**(2): p. 199–212.
13. Visser, S.N., *et al.*, *Trends in the parent-report of health care provider-diagnosed and medicated attention-deficit/hyperactivity disorder: United States, 2003–2011.* Journal of the American Academy of Child & Adolescent Psychiatry, 2014. **53**(1): p. 34–46.
14. Visser, S.N., *et al.*, *Vital signs: national and state-specific patterns of attention deficit/ hyperactivity disorder treatment among insured children aged 2–5 years — United States, 2008–2014.* Morbidity and Mortality Weekly Report, 2016. **65**(17): p. 443–450.
15. Chai, G., *et al.*, *Trends of Outpatient Prescription Drug Utilization in US Children, 2002–2010.* Pediatrics, 2012. **130**(1): p. 23.
16. Qato, D.M., *et al.*, *Prescription Medication Use Among Children and Adolescents in the United States.* Pediatrics, 2018. **142**(3): p. e20181042.

17. Cohen, E., *et al.*, *High-Expenditure Pharmaceutical Use Among Children in Medicaid.* Pediatrics, 2017. **140**(3): p. e20171095.
18. Elliott, C., *Better than well: American medicine meets the American dream*. 2004: WW Norton & Company.
19. Smith, M., *Hyperactive Around the World? The History of ADHD in Global Perspective.* Social History of Medicine, 2017. **30**(4): p. 767–787.
20. Hoshen, M.B., *et al.*, *Stimulant use for ADHD and relative age in class among children in Israel.* Pharmacoepidemiology and Drug Safety, 2016. **25**(6): p. 652–660.
21. Ophir, Y., *Evidence that the Diagnosis of ADHD Does Not Reflect a Chronic Bio-Medical Disease.* Ethical Human Psychology and Psychiatry, 2022. **23**(2).
22. International Narcotics Control Board, *Psychotropic Substances Statistics for 2018 Assessments of Annual Medical and Scientific Requirements*. 2019, https://www.incb.org/documents/Psychotropics/technical-publications/2019/PSY_Technical_Publication_2019.pdf: United Nations — Vienna.
23. International Narcotics Control Board, *Psychotropic Substances Statistics for 2019 Assessments of Annual Medical and Scientific Requirements for 2021*. 2020, https://www.incb.org/documents/Psychotropics/technical-publications/2020/20-06957_Psychotropics_2020_ebook.pdf: United Nations - Vienna.

“

“Psychostimulant compounds are the most widely used medications for the management of ADHD symptoms. Despite their name, these medications do not work by increasing stimulation of the person. Instead, they help important networks of nerve cells in the brain to communicate more effectively with each other. Between 70–80 percent of children with ADHD respond positively to these medications... For some, the benefits are extraordinary; for others, medication is quite helpful; and for still others, the results are more modest.

Attention span, impulsivity and on-task behavior often improve, especially in structured environments. Some children also demonstrate improvements in frustration tolerance, compliance and even handwriting. Relationships with parents, peers and teachers may also improve... Hundreds of controlled studies involving more than 6,000 children, adolescents and adults have been conducted to determine the effects of psychostimulant medications — far more research evidence than is available for virtually any other medication.”

Children and Adults with ADHD (CHADD). *Managing Medication*. Retrieved in November, 2021, from CHADD's webpage [1].

Chapter 8
Are stimulant medications effective in the short term?

If so many children are treated with stimulant medications, they must be highly effective, are they not? Well, if you ask CHADD, as well as multiple other organizations, health officials, and consortiums, the efficacy of stimulant medications — the treatment of choice for Attention Deficit Hyperactivity Disorder (ADHD) (Chapter 7) — has been proven, beyond a shadow of a doubt, in decades of medical research [e.g., 2, 3]. However, when we start to dig a bit further into the available studies, the bright efficacy sand becomes pretty muddy. In Chapter 9, I will target the long-term (and less researched) clinical value of daily usage of stimulant medications, but first, let's examine the validity of the 'easy' and allegedly proven claim that ADHD medications are effective for most children in the short term.

In order to measure the efficacy of any medication, researchers typically conduct experiments (preferably, double blinded, Randomized Controlled Trials) that compare desirable outcomes of at least two groups, one that receives the investigated medication and one that receives a placebo, treatment as usual, or no treatment at all. To examine the duration of the efficacy of the drug, researchers track the performance/improvements of these two, experimental and control, groups, over weeks, months, or years. Notably, in the field of ADHD medications, the vast majority of the "hundreds of controlled studies involving more than 6,000 children, adolescents and adults" mentioned in the opening quote of this chapter [1], lasted only a few weeks, typically between 14 and 49 days [4]. Indeed, the results of these studies usually indicate some reduction in ADHD-related symptoms, but this reduction has not been proven to have clinically valued and sustainable consequences. The National Institute for Health and Care Excellence in the United Kingdom, for example, an organization that supports the use of ADHD medications, did not find evidence for clinical improvements in patients' overall "quality of life" or "any of the important outcomes", except for (short-term) general behavioral improvement and a significant reduction in hyperactivity and inattention symptoms [5, pp. 114-122, 154]. Moreover, a large literature review and meta-analysis by the Cochrane organization that targeted 185 randomized clinical trials, showed that even the straightforward improvement in ADHD symptoms is temporary, minor, and unreliable [4].

If you are unfamiliar with the Cochrane organization (like I was before entering this confusing field), now is a good time to become acquainted with it, especially today, following the medical-scientific uncertainties of the COVID-19 pandemic. The Cochrane organization is a non-profit, voluntary organization comprising scientists and health professionals from 130 countries who are committed to conducting and disseminating high quality and unbiased research. Their goal is to enable people to make medical decisions based on reliable information that is not tainted by conflicts of interest. While even the Cochrane does not always manage to withstand the pressures of the pharmaceutical companies [6], its publications have a unique scientific value. Now, returning to the issue at hand, the literature review and meta-analysis conducted by the Cochrane organization revealed that schoolteachers tend to report behavioral and symptomatic improvements in children who have taken ADHD medications (in this case, methylphenidate). However, the Cochrane researchers also noted that this improvement typically has very little clinical significance for the children themselves [4]. In fact, only three randomized trials (1.6%) documented (small) improvements in the quality of life of the child, as reported by parents in the Child Health Questionnaire [7]. Notably, these studies were judged to be unreliable by the Cochrane researchers (primarily due to methodological failures, selective reporting of results, and conflicts of interest); but even if they were reliable, the average magnitude of their reported quality of life effects was 8 points (on a scale that ranges from 0 to 100), only 1 point higher than the recommended cutoff point for minimal clinically valued improvement [4].

In contrast to the opening quotation of this chapter, the real (short-term) benefits of the medications seem quite modest, and mainly school-related. The medications may improve compliance behavior in school, but they usually do not improve valuable cognitive or emotional skills. This limited clinical value of the medications is also evident in the way people perceive the efficacy of the medications. In my own research (see Chapters 2 and 3), I have noticed that participants almost never use ADHD medications for managing other aspects of life that are not school-related, such as emotional or social functioning [8].

Surprisingly, the very limited clinical value of the medications corresponds with long-standing findings by Prof. Barkley himself (Introduction). Early in his career, when ADHD children were called hyperkinetic children, Barkley noted that "the major effect of the stimulants appears to be an improvement in classroom manageability rather than academic performance" [9, p. 85]. Relying on a literature review that integrated "more objective measures", as he said, Barkley "revealed few positive short-term or long-term drug effects", which could be attributed simply, **in his view**, "to better attention during testing". Although teachers typically report of significant improvements, there is usually no objective difference between treated and untreated children with respect to academic requirements, such as reading, spelling, and math. Stimulant medications, he concluded, "are not able to influence those etiologic factors, other than over activity and inattentiveness, which predispose hyperkinetic children toward school difficulties".

This last conclusion corresponds with a study that was published by Barkley a year later, which showed that hyperactive boys who were treated with Methylphenidate are more compliant to their mothers (compared with a placebo group), but also demonstrated less initiative and were less responsive to their communication efforts [10]. In other words, the medications seem to make children more obedient and 'calm' (see Chapter 10 for more details); however, they do not seem to have significant impact, even if on a short-term basis, on the child's academic performance. And they definitely do not improve the overall quality of life of the child, which is said to be impaired because of the real "brain deficit" (Part One).

At this point, we are ready to move on to the more important, long-term efficacy of the medications (Chapter 9), but first, I wish to propose three reasons why so many 'boots' on the clinical and educational ground believe that the medications are effective, despite their limited value discussed above. My *first hypothesis* is that the initiation of the pharmacological intervention could trigger a somewhat euphoric moment. As introduced in the previous chapter, the biochemical impact of the medications is not fundamentally different from the impact of other non-medical, powerful, and illicit amphetamines, and the initial effects on the child can be dramatic. The child is suddenly performing tasks that previously were felt to be impossible, the teacher marvels at the incredible change and rushes to call the parents to tell them about the miracle that has just occurred ("it's unbelievable, it's as if he's a different child"), and the parents, sometimes, for the first time, can feel proud and, more importantly relieved (their sigh of relief is heartbreaking). This feeling, as if the cork has finally been popped, that the problem is solved, and that the child's true potential can finally be revealed, is a powerful and exciting sensation. But this feeling is equally dangerous, because it is addictive (psychologically) and because it disregards the fact that this "different child" is, in fact, a child who is under the influence of chemical substances. Like most other drugs, the desired magical effect of these substances dissipates within 4–12 hours [11] and the original 'symptoms' return, sometimes in an augmented level, through a rebound effect (Chapters 9 and 10). Over time, compensatory brain mechanisms start to operate and the initial intense response fades (Chapter 11). Consequently, the child must take the medication over and over again in order to achieve the same miraculous and exciting effect that was achieved at the first time. However, as will be shown in the next chapter, to the disappointment of everyone involved, this effect is typically unlikely to reoccur.

My *second hypothesis* is that, like many other medications, the pharmacological intervention for ADHD activates a strong placebo response — an improvement in symptoms that is due, not to the active ingredient of the medication, but rather to the expectation for such an improvement, or the behavioral conditioning that occurred during the first few times of the medication usage. The placebo response is so strong that it is able to improve people's performance on objective Continuous Performance Tests (CPTs), such as the TOVA assessment [12], as well as 'real' clinical symptoms of ADHD (27.6% improvement), as measured by validated scales, such as the Conners rating scale [13]. The boots on the ground (e.g., at school) can therefore easily confuse this placebo response with the effects of the active ingredient in the medication. This is precisely the reason why randomized controlled trials were introduced in the first place. Many times, results from randomized controlled trials indicate an improvement in the experimental group, following the administration of the active ingredient, but a similar or partial improvement also appears in the control group which was given a placebo.

My *third hypothesis* concerns natural improvement. As mentioned in Chapter 3, ADHD symptoms tend to attenuate over time, probably due to the fact that the child's brain matures and his/her cognitive functions improve [14, 15]. As long as the child does not suffer a pervasive cognitive impairment (e.g., Intellectual Disability), there is good reason to assume that ADHD-related behaviors will subside through the years. This is yet another reason why we ought to conduct longitudinal controlled experiments — to rule out this confounding effect of natural improvement. Similar to the placebo effect discussed above, we see in many comparative studies that the control group demonstrates a natural improvement, even when no treatment is given to the participants. This improvement may occur as a result of a common phenomenon known as *regression toward the mean*, but also as a result of the simple fact that the child grows older (Chapter 3).

And yet, despite these hypothetical alternative explanations, there are, of course, quite a few studies that have reported statistically significant short-term benefits of the medications, using acceptable research designs; otherwise, we would not have entered this medication maze in the first place. Nevertheless, the findings from these studies should be interpreted very carefully. Not only did the Cochrane review indicate that the documented short-term benefits were minor, it also suggested that these (minor) benefits are likely to be exaggerated unjustifiably, considering the biased nature of most of the available studies (Chapter 12). The authors of the Cochrane review found that the vast majority of the studies were of poor scientific quality and with a high risk for a significant bias, in which the benefits of the medication were overestimated, while its adverse outcomes were minimized unjustifiably [4]. Thus, we must treat the (minor) improvement reported in clinical research with great skepticism and caution and prioritize high-quality longitudinal research that could shed light on the real, long-term value of stimulant use. The next chapter is dedicated exactly to this type of research, that is: the few studies that have examined the long-term efficacy of stimulant medications for ADHD.

References

1. CHADD, *Managing Medication.* Retreived in November 2021, CHADD: Children and Adults with ADHD, 4221 Forbes Blvd, Suite 270, Lanham, MD, 20706. Last retrieved on November 16, 2021 from: https://chadd.org/for-parents/managing-medication/.
2. National Institute for Health and Care Excellence, *Attention deficit hyperactivity disorder (update) [C] Evidence reviews for pharmacological efficacy and sequencing pharmacological treatment* 2018, Last retrieved on August 20, 2021 from: https://www.nice.org.uk/guidance/ng87/evidence/c-pharmacological-efficacy-and-sequencing-pdf-4783686303.
3. Kooij, J.J.S., *et al., Updated European Consensus Statement on diagnosis and treatment of adult ADHD.* European Psychiatry, 2019. **56**: p. 14–34.
4. Storebø, O.J., *et al., Methylphenidate for attention-deficit/hyperactivity disorder in children and adolescents: Cochrane systematic review with meta-analyses and trial sequential analyses of randomised clinical trials.* Bmj, 2015. **351**.
5. National Institute for Health and Care Excellence, *Attention deficit hyperactivity disorder (update) [C] Evidence reviews for pharmacological efficacy and sequencing pharmacological treatment.* 2018, Last retrieved on August 20, 2021 from: https://www.nice.org.uk/guidance/ng87/evidence/c-pharmacological-efficacy-and-sequencing-pdf-4783686303.
6. Howick, J., *Exploring the asymmetrical relationship between the power of finance bias and evidence.* Perspectives in biology and medicine, 2019. **62**(1): p. 159–187.

7. Rentz, A.M., *et al.*, *Psychometric validation of the child health questionnaire (CHQ) in a sample of children and adolescents with attention-deficit/hyperactivity disorder.* Quality of Life Research, 2005. **14**(3): p. 719–734.
8. Ophir, Y., *Evidence that the Diagnosis of ADHD Does Not Reflect a Chronic Bio-Medical Disease.* Ethical Human Psychology and Psychiatry, 2022. p. **23–2**.
9. Barkley, R.A. and C.E. Cunningham, *Do stimulant drugs improve the academic performance of hyperkinetic children? A review of outcome studies.* Clinical Pediatrics, 1978. **17**(1): p. 85–92.
10. Barkley, R.A. and C.E. Cunningham, *The effects of methylphenidate on the mother-child interactions of hyperactive children.* Archives of General Psychiatry, 1979. **36**(2): p. 201–208.
11. Wolraich, M.L. and M.A. Doffing, *Pharmacokinetic Considerations in the Treatment of Attention-Deficit Hyperactivity Disorder with Methylphenidate.* CNS Drugs, 2004. **18**(4): p. 243–250.
12. Rotem, A., *et al.*, *The Placebo Response in Adult ADHD as Objectively Assessed by the TOVA Continuous Performance Test.* Journal of Attention Disorders, 2020: p. 1087054719897819.
13. Ben-Sheetrit, J., *et al.*, *Characterizing the Placebo Response in Adults With ADHD.* Journal of Attention Disorders, 2020. **24**(3): p. 425–433.
14. Doidge, N., *The brain that changes itself: Stories of personal triumph from the frontiers of brain science.* 2007: Penguin.
15. Rubin, B.P., *Changing brains: The emergence of the field of adult neurogenesis.* BioSocieties, 2009. **4**(4): p. 407–424.

“

“How medication works? Medication does not cure ADHD; when effective, it eases ADHD symptoms during the time it is active. Thus, it is not like an antibiotic that may cure a bacterial infection, but more like eyeglasses that help to improve vision only during the time the eyeglasses are actually worn.”

Children and Adults with ADHD (CHADD). *Medication Management.* Last retrieved on November 16, 2021, from CHADD's webpage [1].

Chapter 9

Are stimulant medications effective in the long term?

For the purpose of the discussion in this chapter, let's assume that medications for Attention Deficit Hyperactivity Disorder (ADHD) do have some clinical value in the short term (a problematic assumption as described in Chapter 8), and ask: What will become of treated children in the future, if and when they decide to stop using their medications? Will the achieved short-term benefits last over time or will they fade? Alternatively, we must ask: What will become of treated children who adhere to their recommended medical plan and use stimulant medications for prolonged periods? After all, ADHD children are said to suffer from a chronic and dangerous brain disorder (Introduction) that should be managed medically throughout their entire development, including adulthood [2]. Medication, as explicitly admitted by CHADD's authors, "does not cure ADHD". The medication "helps regulate the symptoms", as written in the official medication package insert (i.e., the patient leaflet) of the popular medication of Ritalin, "but [it] does not cure" (Figure 3, Chapter 10). It should therefore be used constantly, "like eyeglasses that help to improve vision only during the time the eyeglasses are actually worn" [1]. Unfortunately, these central questions of the current chapter have no reassuring answers.

Longitudinal efficacy

Even strong proponents of the pharmacological treatment for ADHD typically acknowledge the fact that, to date, there is no convincing evidence that the medications are effective in the long term [e.g., 3]. All these years, since the establishment of ADHD in 1980, physicians and researchers have known, of course, about the absence of evidence for long-term efficacy. In 1992, the National Institute of Mental Health (NIMH) even decided to take action and conduct a longitudinal Randomized Controlled Trial (RCT) — the gold-standard research in medical science — to resolve this open question once and for all. This seminal study was named the 'Multimodal Treatment of ADHD' study, or in short, the MTA study, and to this day, it is considered the highest quality research on this matter, due to its solid *internal validity* (Box 1, Chapter 1).

The first results from the MTA study, which were published 14 months after its initiation, provided proponents of the medications with a cause for celebration. The medications seemed so successful at reducing symptoms of ADHD that there was no need for any additional intervention, such as behavioral therapy — a form of non-pharmacological treatment that was provided to participants alongside the medications in one of the experimental arms of the study [4]. However, with time, the premature celebrations have turned to funeral cries. By 24 months, the benefits of the medications decreased significantly [5], and "by 36 months, the earlier advantage of having had 14 months of the medication algorithm was no longer apparent" [6, p. 989]. Unexpectedly, a three-year follow-up of the MTA study revealed that "24- to 36-month medication use was a significant marker… not of beneficial outcome, but of deterioration. That is, participants using medication in the 24- to 36-month period actually showed increased symptomatology during that interval relative to those not taking medication" (page 996).

Notice that I presented the above findings in their original wording so readers will know that the unbelievable conclusions from the MTA study are not my subjective interpretation of its findings. In fact, most of the authors of this last study [the 3-year follow-up study; 6] were members of the original MTA Cooperative Group [5], and some of them are considered as the 'big names' of the field. Prof. Keith Conners, "the father of ADHD" (Introduction), is only one example. Another noteworthy name in this context is Prof. Peter Jensen, the first author of this 3-year follow-up. Prof. Jensen served as the head of child psychiatry at the NIMH, and he was the one who led the writing of the 14-months report of the MTA study. As you might recall from the Introduction, Prof. Jensen was also one of the prominent supporters of the pharmacological treatment in the NIMH Consensus Development Conference, back in 1998.

A second noteworthy leader of the MTA study is Prof. James Swanson, the director of the Child Development Center at the University of California who had also contributed to the Consensus Development Conference. "The findings of these secondary articles" three years following the beginning of the MTA study, writes Swanson, together with Jensen and multiple other key researchers in the field, "were not consistent with some expectations about medication effects that were generally accepted by many of the field's investigators and clinicians in 2007" [7, p. 11]. A close reading of their conclusions paper from 2008 (titled: Evidence, Interpretation, and Qualification From Multiple Reports of Long-Term Outcomes in the MTA study of Children with ADHD) suggests that the researchers tried to 'save' their original consensual expectations using post-hoc rationalizations, but they could not find any reasonable explanation that aligns with the favorable beliefs regarding the efficacy of the medications: "selection bias was not shown to account for the loss of relative superiority of medication over time; there was no evidence for "catch-up" growth; early treatment with medication did not protect against later adverse outcomes" [7, p. 11].

As time went by, the promises of the medications continued to be shattered by science. Six and eight years later, the medicated group showed no advantage over the unmedicated control group, neither in reducing ADHD symptomatology nor in improving academic performance [8]. A final nail in the coffin of the medication narrative was revealed in the MTA-based article that reported of zero positive effects of ADHD medications (which were taken in childhood) in adulthood [9].

In Chapter 12, I discuss how it is possible that the public is unaware of these groundbreaking findings, but it is important to acknowledge here that the MTA study is not the only place where readers can get a glimpse of truth regarding the efficacy of the medications. Similar findings to the MTA results are hidden, for example, in a recent meta-analysis on functional outcomes of medication use [10]. Although the leading narrative of this meta-analysis is highly pro-medication, the calculated overall effect of the medications on academic performance (as measured by continuous scales) was found to be neutral (for more intriguing information about this study, see the last section of this chapter and Chapter 12). In other words, there is considerable data that undermine the notion that medication use can lead to academic improvements over time, let alone symptom reduction or other cognitive and emotional benefits.

Longitudinal reverse efficacy

Not only did the MTA study not find any benefits to medication use, but six years after the onset of the study, medication use predicted worse ADHD-related symptoms as well as worse Oppositional Defiant Disorder symptoms and overall functioning impairments [8]. Apparently, the major conclusion from this 'super study', the highest quality longitudinal research available, was that the longer children use ADHD medications, the worse their symptoms and functioning is expected to be over time!

Similar conclusions have been drawn from prospective longitudinal studies conducted in Canada and Australia as well. A naturalistic study conducted in the province of Quebec found a deterioration in academic performance, including a decline in math scores, following a public health policy change which led to an increase in the use of ADHD medications [11]. Another large-scale study conducted in Western Australia, 'the Raine Study', found that the use of ADHD medications over time was associated with poor school performance and increased risk to be identified as an academic failure [12]. Essentially, these studies provide preliminary evidence for the notion that medications for ADHD can **produce** ADHD-like symptoms when they are used for prolonged periods (see Chapter 11, for the brain mechanism that might underlie this notion).

Longitudinal protection

Considering the dubious long-term efficacy in symptom reduction, researchers (backed by pharma companies) turned to argue that the medications have a critical protective role against future dangers and adverse events. This argument consists of two subclaims. The first claim (according to the deterministic biomedical view of ADHD) is that ADHD is bound to increase the risk for multiple adverse outcomes, including, for example, car accidents, substance abuse, and incarcerations (Chapter 4). The second claim is that regular usage of stimulant medications can protect against these expected dangers. The aforementioned meta-analysis on functional outcomes of medication use, for example, concluded in 2020 that ADHD medications were proven to reduce the risk of a wide-ranging set of adverse events associated with ADHD [10]. Correspondingly, previous studies suggested that medications can protect against injuries and accidents [13], delinquency [14], drug abuse [15], suicide behaviors [16], and even highly infectious diseases, such as the COVID-19 acute respiratory syndrome [17].

But how accurate are these claims? Part One of the book has already refuted the deterministic biomedical view about ADHD (e.g., Chapter 6) and shown that ADHD does not meet the danger criterion of psychiatric diagnosis (Chapter 4). ADHD does not cause premature death (while comorbid disorders and medications might do) and the non-fatal dangers that are claimed to result from the disorder are rare, unreliable, and, in too many cases, presented in a biased manner. Of course, some individuals take more risks than others [18], but there is a huge gap between this plain interpersonal difference and the claim that ADHD is a dangerous condition [e.g., 19]. The dangerous component is not part of the diagnostic criteria in ADHD [20], it does not apply to young children, and to the best of my knowledge, it has never been associated with ADHD in a direct, causal relationship (for a comprehensive rebuttal of the danger intimidations, see Chapter 4). On the contrary, it is much more likely that we are witnessing the problematic phenomenon, known as *disease mongering* [21, 22], whereby pharmaceutical companies and their representatives artificially exaggerate the prevalence, severity, and dangers of medical conditions (for more details, see Chapter 12).

Now, let's return to the aforementioned updated meta-analysis [10] and investigate the validity of the second claim, according to which medications were proven to protect against the (exaggerated and unreliable) dangers of ADHD. Apparently, despite the authors' straightforward assertion in the abstract section that the findings "suggest that ADHD medication treatments are associated with decreases in the risks for a wide range of ADHD-associated functional outcomes" (page 21), the picture that arises from the actual findings of this meta-analysis is completely different [23]. First, the overall 'protective' effects of the medications on suicidality and on traumatic brain injury relied on two studies only. They suffered from significant heterogeneity and most importantly, they were **not** significant. Second, the overall effects of the medications on substance use and on criminality also relied on two studies and were also **not** significant. Third, the only potential significant overall effect on accidents and injuries that relied on several studies ($N = 6$), suffered from a significant heterogeneity, which challenges the interpretation of the effect and perhaps even explains why the aforementioned consumer leaflet of Ritalin instructs its users to "exercise caution when driving" (Figure 3, Chapter 10). Finally, even the straightforward effect on the continuous variables of academic performances, as mentioned earlier in this chapter, was neutral.

What then can explain this narrative 'spin', in which the abstract section of the meta-analysis presents a completely different picture than its actual findings? At first glance, there seems to be no motive for such a discrepancy, as "all authors report no potential conflicts of interest to disclose above the ones reported in the financial disclosures" [10, p. 29]. However, when stubborn readers manage to read the financial disclosures section (a section that is displayed at the end of the manuscript, after the long list of references), they suddenly realize that four senior researchers reported of relationships with the pharma industry. These inherent conflicts of interest may also explain why the authors chose to omit their findings regarding the existence of a publication bias. They specifically stated that they "used the Egger method to assess for publication biases" [10, p. 22], but they only provided this crucial information in their last analysis on academic performance (which, as mentioned above, produced a neutral overall effect).[1] Thus, when examined together — the relationships with the pharma industry, the omissions of publication bias results, and the mostly non-significant, un-replicated, and heterogeneous overall effects of the medications — challenge the conclusion of the meta-analysis, as if ADHD medications can decrease the risks for "a wide range of ADHD-associated functional outcomes".

Similar spins and distortions were found in the recently published study that warned that ADHD could increase the risk for COVID-19 infections, and that stimulant medications are able to mitigate that risk [17]. Although the authors of this study did not report of conflicts of interest, their study consisted of multiple distortions that do not allow us to trust its conclusions [23]. I discuss the specifics of this study in detail in Chapter 12, but it is important to mention here that my review of this study, together with the health communication researcher, Dr. Yaffa Shir-Raz, yielded seven manipulations and narrative spins designed (even if not intentionally) to convince the reader that ADHD medications can mitigate the risk for COVID-19 infections [23]. Not only that the authors of this study failed to provide reliable proof for their claim regarding the protective role of the medications, they also completely ignored this claim in their following study on severe COVID-19 outcomes, which was published less than a year later, in the same journal [24]. Needless to say that this secondary study, did not include the required stratification to treated and untreated participants [25]. With so many unexplainable distortions, it is my view that these two COVID-19 studies are essentially part of the everlasting disease mongering efforts in ADHD (Chapter 12). In this way, they join the many other biased studies that chose to exaggerate the efficacy of the

---

[1] The small number of studies in this subcategory ("academic outcomes") raises the speculation that the Egger test was actually conducted on the entire set of studies presented in this meta-analysis, and that its location within this subcategory is accidental. However, if this speculation is true, then the overall effect of the entire set of studies should have been presented in the article as well. After all, such an Egger test can only be conducted within the context of an inclusive meta-analysis that takes into account the entire set of studies — an inclusive meta-analysis that, regrettably, was not reported in the article. In response to my query on this matter, the corresponding author of this article [10] replied that he is "unable to provide with any additional information" beyond the information given in the published article. I have also tried to contact the first author of this article, but she did not reply to my query.

medications [26], probably under the influence of the pharmaceutical industry [27].

Fortunately (in my opinion), real-life observations suggest that the general public usually does not 'buy' the risks that are marketed to parents and children through such disease mongering practices. As mentioned in Chapter 8, only very few people (2–3%) use ADHD medications for non-school related purposes, such as emotional or social functioning. Most patients, children and adults, use ADHD medications very selectively, mainly during school/college time, to improve school-related performance. Similarly, most parents avoid giving ADHD medications to their children outside of the school context [28]. Surprisingly, these consumer behaviors are not detached from the more formal instructions of the official patient leaflet of the popular medication of Ritalin, as approved by the Israel Ministry of Health (Figure 3, Chapter 10). Unlike "eyeglasses that help to improve vision" [1], the consumer leaflet explicitly dictates that, "the doctor may tell you to stop taking Ritalin for certain period of time (e.g., every weekend or school vacations)". Notice that the school-related example presented in the parentheses appears in the original text of the leaflet, in contrast to the ruling consensus that the chronic 'brain deficit' should be managed medically every day (Introduction). In other words, even consensual bodies, such as the Israeli Ministry of Health, recognize that the medications (that work for several hours only), are not crucially needed to protect against daily or future dangers.

Medication efficacy in a nutshell

Despite the existence of "hundreds of studies" on stimulant medications [29], the information presented in this chapter as well as the previous one (Chapter 8), undermines the claim that continuous medication use has sustainable and valuable positive outcomes. Even if some of these hundreds of studies are not distorted and are not under the influence of the pharma industry (Chapter 12), the vast majority of them are of very poor scientific quality and their duration rarely extends beyond several weeks (Chapter 8). Notably, the very few studies that are of high quality, such as the longitudinal and controlled MTA study, depict a completely different picture from the one described by the biomedical consensus. The medications have very little (if any) clinical value for patients in the short term, and they probably have zero value in the long term. On the contrary, there is now accumulative evidence that stimulant medications increase ADHD-like symptoms and functional impairments. Unfortunately, not only do medications not protect against future risks, such as drug use or criminal activities, they also put the user at a great risk for multiple dangers, as will be shown in great detail in the following chapters (Chapters 10 and 11).

References

1. CHADD, *Medication Management.* Retrieved on November, 2021, Children and Adults with Attention-Deficit/Hyperactivity Disorder (CHADD). Last retrieved on November 16, 2021, from: https://chadd.org/for-adults/medication-management/.
2. Kooij, J.J.S., *et al., Updated European Consensus Statement on diagnosis and treatment of adult ADHD.* European Psychiatry, 2019. **56**: p. 14–34.
3. Chang, Z., *et al., Risks and Benefits of Attention-Deficit/Hyperactivity Disorder Medication on Behavioral and Neuropsychiatric Outcomes: A Qualitative Review of Pharmacoepidemiology Studies Using Linked Prescription Databases.* Biological Psychiatry, 2019. **86**(5): p. 335–343.
4. MTA Cooperative Group, *A 14-month randomized clinical trial of treatment strategies for attention-deficit/hyperactivity disorder.* Archives of General Psychiatry, 1999. **56**(12): p. 1073–1086.
5. MTA Cooperative Group, *National Institute of Mental Health Multimodal Treatment Study of ADHD follow-up: 24-month outcomes of treatment strategies for attention-deficit/hyperactivity disorder.* Pediatrics, 2004. **113**(4): p. 754–761.
6. Jensen, P.S., *et al., 3-year follow-up of the NIMH MTA study.* Journal of the American Academy of Child & Adolescent Psychiatry, 2007. **46**(8): p. 989–1002.

7. Swanson, J., *et al.*, *Evidence, interpretation, and qualification from multiple reports of long-term outcomes in the Multimodal Treatment Study of Children with ADHD (MTA) Part I: Executive Summary.* Journal of Attention Disorders, 2008. **12**(1): p. 4–14.
8. Molina, B.S.G., *et al.*, *The MTA at 8 years: prospective follow-up of children treated for combined-type ADHD in a multisite study.* Journal of the American Academy of Child & Adolescent Psychiatry, 2009. **48**(5): p. 484–500.
9. Swanson, J.M., *et al.*, *Young adult outcomes in the follow-up of the multimodal treatment study of attention-deficit/hyperactivity disorder: symptom persistence, source discrepancy, and height suppression.* Journal of Child Psychology and Psychiatry, 2017. **58**(6): p. 663–678.
10. Boland, H., *et al.*, *A literature review and meta-analysis on the effects of ADHD medications on functional outcomes.* Journal of Psychiatric Research, 2020. **123**: p. 21–30.
11. Currie, J., M. Stabile, and L. Jones, *Do stimulant medications improve educational and behavioral outcomes for children with ADHD?* Journal of Health Economics, 2014. **37**: p. 58–69.
12. Whitely, M., *The rise and fall of ADHD child prescribing in Western Australia: Lessons and implications.* Australian & New Zealand Journal of Psychiatry, 2012. **46**(5): p. 400–403.
13. Chen, V.C.-H., *et al.*, *The association between methylphenidate treatment and the risk for fracture among young ADHD patients: A nationwide population-based study in Taiwan.* PloS one, 2017. **12**(3).
14. Mohr-Jensen, C., *et al.*, *Attention-Deficit/Hyperactivity Disorder in Childhood and Adolescence and the Risk of Crime in Young Adulthood in a Danish Nationwide Study.* Journal of the American Academy of Child & Adolescent Psychiatry, 2019. **58**(4): p. 443–452.
15. Chang, Z., *et al.*, *Stimulant ADHD medication and risk for substance abuse.* Journal of Child Psychology and Psychiatry, 2014. **55**(8): p. 878–885.
16. Liang, S.H.-Y., *et al.*, *Suicide risk reduction in youths with attention-deficit/hyperactivity disorder prescribed methylphenidate: a Taiwan nationwide population-based cohort study.* Research in Developmental Disabilities, 2018. **72**: p. 96–105.
17. Merzon, E., *et al.*, *ADHD as a Risk Factor for Infection With Covid-19.* Journal of Attention Disorders, 2020. **25**(13): p. 1783–1790.

18. Pollak, Y., *et al.*, *The role of parental monitoring in mediating the link between adolescent ADHD symptoms and risk-taking behavior.* Journal of Attention Disorders, 2020. **24**(8): p. 1141–1147.
19. Vaa, T., *ADHD and relative risk of accidents in road traffic: A meta-analysis.* Accident Analysis & Prevention, 2014. **62**: p. 415–425.
20. APA, *Diagnostic and Statistical Manual of Mental Disorders (DSM-5®).* 2013: American Psychiatric Association.
21. Blasco-Fontecilla, H., *Medicalization, wish-fulfilling medicine, and disease mongering: toward a brave new world?* Revista Clinica Espanola, 2014. **214**(2): p. 104–107.
22. Wolinsky, H., *Disease mongering and drug marketing.* EMBO reports, 2005. **6**(7): p. 612–614.
23. Ophir, Y. and Y. Shir-Raz, *Manipulations and Spins in Attention Disorders Research: The Case of ADHD and COVID-19.* Ethical Human Psychology and Psychiatry, 2020. **22**: p. 98–113.
24. Merzon, E., *et al.*, *The Association between ADHD and the Severity of COVID-19 Infection.* Journal of Attention Disorders, 2021. **26**(4): p. 491–501.
25. Ophir, Y. and Y. Shir-Raz, *Discrepancies in Studies on ADHD and COVID-19 Raise Concerns Regarding the Risks of Stimulant Treatments During an Active Pandemic.* Accepted Manuscript. Ethical Human Psychology and Psychiatry.
26. Storebø, O.J., *et al.*, *Methylphenidate for attention deficit hyperactivity disorder (ADHD) in children and adolescents–assessment of adverse events in non-randomised studies.* Cochrane Database of Systematic Reviews, 2018(5).
27. Whitaker, R. and L. Cosgrove, *Psychiatry under the influence: Institutional corruption, social injury, and prescriptions for reform.* 2015: Springer.
28. Ophir, Y., *Evidence that the Diagnosis of ADHD Does Not Reflect a Chronic Bio-Medical Disease.* Ethical Human Psychology and Psychiatry, 2022. **23–2**.
29. CHADD, *Managing Medication.* Retreived on November 2021, CHADD: Children and Adults with ADHD, 4221 Forbes Blvd, Suite 270, Lanham, MD, 20706. Last retrieved on November 16, 2021 from: https://chadd.org/for-parents/managing-medication/.

"

"ADHD Medication Safe, Experts Say: Parents of kids with attention-deficit hyperactivity disorder (ADHD) face a tough choice: whether to medicate their children or not... It's a touchy subject, and it got even thornier after recent reports linked popular ADHD drugs to increased health risks, especially risks for heart problems. But the top experts at the American Academy of Pediatrics, as well as at other professional groups for ADHD and cardiology experts, say the drugs are safe. These experts have found that heart risks are not increased by treating ADHD any more than the risks for the same rare heart problems in children without ADHD who are not taking ADHD medications. Medications to treat ADHD are effective, and reports of major problems are extremely rare."

Stanford Children's Health. *ADHD Medication Safe, Experts Say.* Last retrieved in November, 2021 from: Lucile Packard Children's Hospital Stanford webpage [1].

Chapter 10
What are the 'non-serious' safety concerns of stimulant use?

Have you ever stopped for a moment to ask why, apart from the MTA study (Chapter 9), there are no other high-quality studies on the long-term efficacy of stimulant medications? Although such studies can be expensive and complex to carry out, they are probably worth the trouble, particularly for the pharmaceutical companies. After all, a high-quality study that will prove that a certain medication has a long-term efficacy could substantially amplify its sales. A preliminary answer to this question may be that longitudinal studies, as shown in the previous chapter, can expose undesirable results (from the perspective of the pharma industry, which typically funds such studies). However, another possible and more alarming answer may be that such high-quality longitudinal experiments would reveal the large proportions of dropouts — that is, the many participants who could not complete the study because they suffered extensive adverse events [2]. Forming additional longitudinal Randomized Controlled Trials (RCTs) might expose serious adverse outcomes of medications for Attention Deficit Hyperactivity Disorder (ADHD) — outcomes that will then be very difficult to minimize or dismiss, because of the high *internal validity* (Box 1, Chapter 1) of such controlled trials.

Consider the MTA study, for example. Apart from the decline in academic performance and the worsening of symptoms, it turned out that prolonged medication usage also had lasting negative effects on the child's development. Children who adhered to their medication plan during childhood grew up to be significantly shorter adults than their ADHD peers who used their medications inconsistently or negligibly [3]. Contrary to prior expectations, the MTA study did not yield evidence for a compensatory growth 'rebound' or 'catch-up' [4], and the final, average height difference (4.7 centimeters) between consistent users and negligible users in adulthood was quite dramatic

[3]. This growth suppression is a well-documented side effect of the medications [2, 5] and even strong proponents of pharmacological treatments acknowledge its existence [6, 7]. The *medication package insert* (i.e., the patient leaflet) of the popular medication of Ritalin, for example — an official source of information that was checked and approved by the Israeli Ministry of Health — justifies the implementation of 'treatment breaks' during weekends and holidays, with an explicit statement according to which such breaks can "help prevent a slow-down in growth that sometimes occurs when children take this medicine for a long time" (Figure 3). Indeed, typical marketing strategies try to minimize this highly established adverse outcome by framing it as a non-serious, mild event. But is it really that mild? After all, whether the impact on the child's growth is due to the daily appetite suppression, or to a more acute and persistent inhibition of growth hormones [6, 8], how can we be sure that this growth impairment is 'only' an aesthetic damage and not a more pervasive slowdown of critical developmental processes, including the developmental processes of the brain itself? Who knows what exactly the growth price entails?

But for those who still view growth suppression as a reasonable developmental price to pay, and for those who trust the "top experts" who insist that "the drugs are safe", as declared in the opening citation of this chapter [1], let us investigate some of the other, dozens of adverse effects of the medications. To my knowledge, all researchers, including the ones who support the use of medications, admit that stimulant medications may trigger a range of unwanted risks. The more accurate question of this chapter (and the following chapter) should therefore **not** be whether stimulant medications are safe, but rather to what extent stimulant medications trigger adverse outcomes, and to what extent the quantity and intensity of these adverse outcomes are substantially lower than their beneficial outcomes. Since the previous chapters have already exposed the very limited (if any) clinical benefit of the medications, especially for the long term (Chapters 8 and 9), we are left mainly with the safety part of this last question: how dangerous and harmful are stimulant medications? The current chapter and the following one provide an overview of the somewhat hidden evidence regarding the adverse outcomes of stimulant medications, starting with the presumably non-serious outcomes (not to startle the dear reader), in this chapter, and continuing with long-term and highly serious outcomes in the next chapter (Chapter 11).

Non-serious outcomes for beginners

Like all psychiatric drugs, the list of adverse outcomes of stimulant medications is quite long, consisting mostly of events that are considered non-serious. But to what extent these events (that occur mostly to children — the main costumers of these medications), are truly 'non-serious', readers can judge for themselves. According to a literature review of 44 studies that investigated the outcomes of methylphenidate (e.g., Ritalin, Concerta), non-serious adverse events may include: restlessness, hyperactivity (no, this is not a mistake), dizziness, nail biting, nightmares, crying, reduced speech, tics, aggressive behaviors, emotional lability, anxiety, and depression [9]. Upon reading this short, and certainly non-exhaustive, list of non-serious events, parents of ADHD children might think to themselves "well, the pharma companies are obligated to mention these side effects, but these effects are ought to be very rare, otherwise they would not have been marketed to children with mundane difficulties". Little do parents know about the actual prevalence of these non-serious events, and it's not their fault. This is the message they receive from consensual health officials: "ADHD medication safe, experts say" [1].

For example, the aforementioned patient leaflet of Ritalin, which was approved by the Israeli Ministry of Health, delivers the following reassuring message: "As with any medicine, use of Ritalin may cause side effects in some users. Do not be alarmed by the list of side effects. **You may not suffer from any of them**" (Figure 3; bold added by Y.O.). Unfortunately, this statement is inaccurate and misleading, as most users of methylphenidate (the active ingredient in Ritalin), would suffer from one or more adverse outcomes [2].

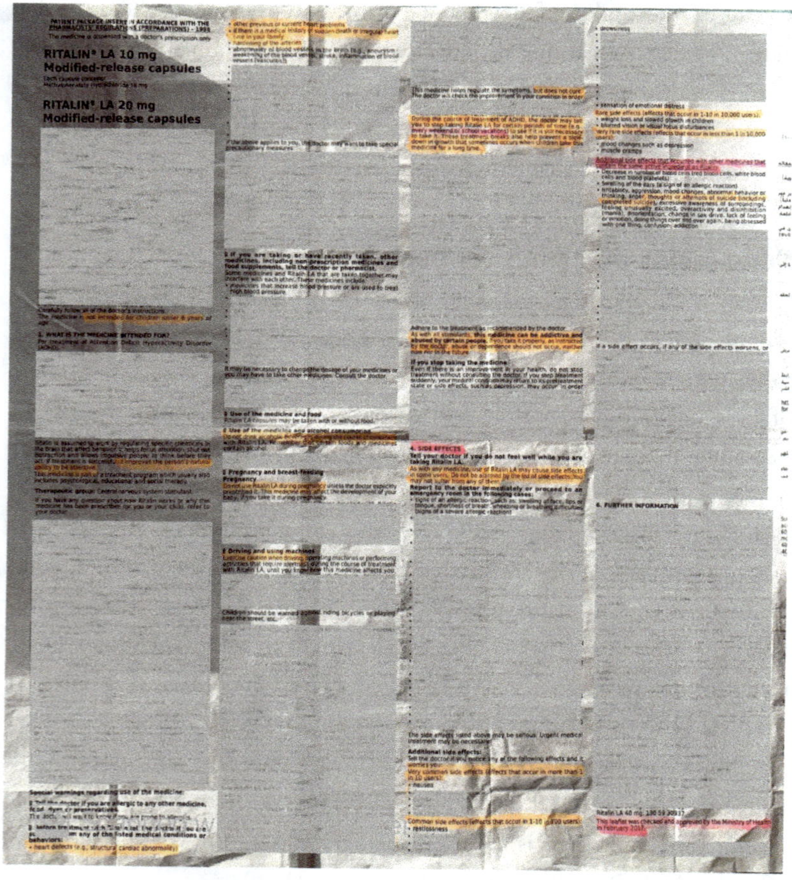

PATIENT PACKAGE INSERT IN ACCORDANCE WITH THE PHARMACISTS' REGULATIONS (PREPARATIONS) - 1986

The medicine is dispensed with a doctor's prescription only

RITALIN® LA 10 mg
Modified-release capsules

RITALIN® LA 20 mg
Modified-release capsules

1. WHAT IS THE MEDICINE INTENDED FOR?

• other previous or current heart problems

• hardening of the arteries

If you are taking or have recently taken, other medicines, including non-prescription medicines and food supplements, tell the doctor or pharmacist.
Some medicines and Ritalin LA that are taken together may interfere with each other. These medicines include:
• medicines that increase blood pressure or are used to treat high blood pressure

It may be necessary to change the dosage of your medicines or you may have to take other medicines. Consult the doctor.

Use of the medicine and food
Ritalin LA capsules may be taken with or without food.

Use of the medicine and alcohol consumption

Pregnancy and breast-feeding

Driving and using machines

4. SIDE EFFECTS

Additional side effects:

6. FURTHER INFORMATION

Figure 3. Medication package insert (patient leaflet) of Ritalin. To maintain 'fare use' of the leaflet, most of its content has been redacted (although public interest dictates that all information about medications will be transparent and available). The specific leaflet in the image "was checked and approved by the Israeli Ministry of Health in February 2017".

This last fact regarding the extremely high prevalence of adverse events is backed by the recent Cochrane review of 260 non-randomized studies [2]. The complete list of adverse outcomes of this review is too long to be included in this chapter (see pages 29–38 in the previous citation), so I will only mention a few representative non-serious events from the first cluster of the 'central nervous system events' (other documented clusters of events are the cardiovascular and respiratory system, gastrointestinal system, musculoskeletal system, which includes height and weight, immune system, urogenital system, and other body systems).

Alarmingly, the percentage of methylphenidate users with affect lability was 29.8%; anxiety was 18.4%; difficulty falling asleep was 17.9%; sadness was 16.8%; anorexia was 16.5%; isolation and lack of interest in others was 15.9%; fingernail biting was 14.3%; increased need to sleep was 11.7%; nightmares was 8.10%; tics was 6.4%; 'zombie-like' demeanor was 5.20%; and depression was 4%. Importantly, this list of non-serious outcomes also included events that could easily be attributed to the disorder itself, as large proportions of users experienced daydreams (35.1%), excessive talking (17.6%), irritability (17.2%), restlessness and agitation (7.40%), and involuntary movements (6.30%). These adverse outcomes correspond with the increase in ADHD-related symptoms found in the experimental group of the MTA study, which was treated with stimulant medications (Chapter 9).

Evidence regarding the high prevalence of adverse outcomes is not confined to impartial reviews, such as the one made by the Cochrane. Barkley himself, the expert that is probably most identified with the consensual biomedical approach (Introduction), reported of high prevalence of non-serious outcomes among an experimental group of children who received methylphenidate, compared to a control group of children who were given a placebo treatment [10]. In some of these non-serious events (e.g., decreased appetite headache, abdominal pain, sleep disorders, and tics), the percentage gap between the experimental and the control groups ranged from 10% to 40%.

Misrepresentations of adverse outcomes

Non-serious events, as can be seen from the previous (selective and short) lists, are by no means uncommon. Yet, for some reason (Chapter 12), the official patient leaflet presents much rosier prevalence estimates of potential adverse outcomes (Figure 3). For example, "restlessness" and "irritability" are said to occur in 1 in 10 users, and "mood changes such as depression" is said to occur in less than 1 in 10,000 users. I therefore decided to inquire about the prevalence of some representative adverse outcomes effects myself. I have asked a sample of 218 Israeli young adults who have used stimulant medications in the past, either as children, or as adults, to complete a close-ended questionnaire that addressed three problematic aspects of medication use: (1) adverse events, (2) signs of medication dependence, and (3) signs of drug abuse [11]. When relating to the first aspect of medication use, that is the question regarding adverse events, I made sure to use the same wording as the official patient leaflet (I only copied eight representative items from the leaflet because the list of adverse events was too long to impose on the participants of the study). I have also taken the liberty to add five additional adverse events that, for some reason, did not appear in the leaflet, but should have been mentioned there, based on my impression from the field and the literature (see Table 3 for the entire list of events measured in the study at hand).

Before presenting my findings, let me first admit that I am not claiming that the results from this explorative study can be generalized 'as-is' to all users of stimulants. The internal validity of the study is inherently limited due to its observational nature and the lack of a designated control group that would have allowed me to scrutinize the exact prevalence rates of the adverse effects of the medications. Yet, considering the available research and especially the aforementioned conclusions from the Cochrane review, I believe that the findings of this study should be taken seriously.

As hypothesized, the study documented multiple adverse events, including serious outcomes (Table 3). The prevalence of almost all the adverse outcomes of the medications was extremely high, including the ones reported "rare" or "very rare" in the patient leaflet. Nonparametric analyses, which were conducted whenever a comparison could be made, showed that all the observed events were significantly and substantially more prevalent than their reported estimates in the patient leaflet. "Mood changes such as depression", for example, was experienced by 66% of the sample, a substantially higher number than the reported "very rare side effect that occur in 1 in 10,000 users" of the leaflet ($\chi^2 = 22463.325$, $p < .0001$). This last outcome, and by no means, mild adverse event, is discussed in length later in this chapter, in the context of the operative mechanism of the medications, but it is important to acknowledge here that stimulant medications have long been suspected to trigger depressive states. The Canadian study mentioned in Chapter 9, for example, showed evidence of a dramatic rise in depression rates among girls following the policy change, which substantially increased the rates of stimulant use in Quebec [12].

Table 3. Perceived adverse side effects of ADHD medications [11]

Adverse effect	Prevalence	Statistical analyses
Very common side effects (effects that occur in more than 1 in 10 users)		
1. Decreased appetite	77.1%	(expected value ≥10%)
Common side effects (effects that occur in 1–10 in 100 users)		
2. Restlessness	42%	$\chi^2 = 251.174$, $p < .0001$ (expected value ≤10%)
3. Headache	32%	$\chi^2 = 123.376$, $p < .0001$ (expected value ≤10%)
4. Excessive sweating	20%	$\chi^2 = 23.23$, $p < .0001$ (expected value ≤10%)
Rare side effects (effects that occur in 1–10 in 10,000 users)		
5. Weight loss	32%	$\chi^2 = 22463.325$, $p < .0001$ (expected value ≤0.1%)
Very rare side effects (effects that occur in less than 1 in 10,000 users)		
6. Mood changes such as depression	66%	$\chi^2 = 950999.782$, $p < .0001$ (expected value ≤0.01%)

(Continued)

Table 3. (*Continued*)

Adverse effect	Prevalence	Statistical analyses
7. Muscle cramps	6.45%	$\chi^2 = 9005.180$, $p < .0001$ (expected value ≤0.01%)
Additional side effects that occurred with other medications that contain the same active ingredient as Ritalin		
8. Thoughts of attempts of suicide	3.2%	Expected value is not reported in the leaflet
Clinically observed side effects that are not listed in the leaflet		
9. Zombie-like sensation, apathy, or a feeling of dissociation	72.5%	
10. Alterations in sense of self — a psychological feeling as if I am not myself	39.4%	
11. Recurrent and disturbing thoughts	31.3%	
12. Thoughts or attempts of self-harm, such as cutting oneself	3.7%	
13. Severe side effects (extreme physical/emotional reactions) that require an immediate cessation of the medications	2.8%	

Note: The adverse effects that were copied from the medication package insert are ordered according to their stated prevalence in the patient leaflet on the left column. The column in the middle shows the actual prevalence that was documented in the study. Nonparametric analyses were conducted whenever a comparison could be made between the documented prevalence and the leaflet prevalence (i.e., some effects/rates of effects were not reported in the patient leaflet).

Aside from these gaps between the leaflet prevalence and the reported prevalence of adverse outcomes, I also discovered high rates of other, adverse events that are not mentioned in the leaflet, including for example: 'zombie-like sensation, apathy, or a feeling of dissociation' (72.5%), 'alterations in the sense of self — a psychological feeling as if I am not myself' (39.4%), and 'recurrent and disturbing thoughts' (31.3%). I was also perturbed to find out that a relatively large number of users (28%) reported that they tried to resist taking the medications as children when told to do so by their adult caregivers. I therefore posit that we can no longer relate to the non-serious outcomes of the medications as mild and rare events. My study, along with the Cochrane review, and multiple other studies that are presented further in this chapter, do not support the popular belief that the medications are harmless. In the next sections, I discuss two very common 'non-serious' adverse outcomes of stimulant medications, which are sometimes interpreted (by adult caregivers) as behavioral improvements, despite their significant negative impact on the child's well-being.

The oppression of the body

One of the most common 'non-serious' outcomes of stimulant medications is a constant feeling of lethargy [13]. A total of 18% of children who used stimulants were described by independent raters (who were blind to the medication status of the child) in a time-worn study, as "tired, withdrawn, listless, depressed, dopey, dazed, subdued, and inactive" [13, p. 1104]. This common reaction has been known to researchers and physicians for decades. Early studies from the 1980s and the 1990s have reported that many children, who were using stimulant medications for their ADHD, exhibited zombie-like behaviors [14] and appeared to external observers as withdrawn, indifferent, and even in shock. In a way, the drug can be seen as a method to oppress spontaneous behaviors. It decreases children's natural curiosity [15] and causes many of them to be apathetic, passive, and submissive [16]. Dr. Leonard Sax had even argued, based on biochemical evidence (see also Chapter 11), that the growing use of ADHD medications is one of the key factors that underlie the wide phenomena of unmotivated children and underachieving adults in America [17]. No wonder that the Cochrane review documented high prevalence of isolation and lack of interest in others, increased need to sleep, zombie-like conduct, and depression [2].

Surprisingly, much of these common reactions are not mentioned in the official patient leaflet presented before (Figure 3). I, of course, have no way of knowing why the familiar zombie-like condition, indifference, and apathy, are not mentioned in the leaflet. I can only suspect that the authors of the leaflet feared that the general public would realize that the desired outcomes of the drug (a decrease in hyperactivity and distracted behaviors) are essentially a major adverse outcome of the drug [18, Ch. 6]. Another example of an attempt to hide this side effect can be seen in a relatively old short-term RCT that promoted the use of methylphenidate among preschool children [19]. Whereas the abstract of the study minimizes the magnitude of the adverse outcomes of the medication, its actual results suggest that **kindergarten children**, who used the medication in high doses, were significantly less interested in other children and significantly less lively than their peers who were not given the medication.

Of course, I am not expecting proponents of the disorder to be aware of all the available research. This is an impossible requirement, which I, myself, do not presume to fulfil (see the Interim Summary of Part One). Yet, in this case, the knowledge has been available to representatives of the biomedical consensus for decades. Barkley himself noticed, back in the 1970s, that the overall level of activity of children who used ADHD medications decreased significantly, and that these children preferred to play alone [20]. I sometimes imagine these medications as heavyweights, which make children more 'calm' through the strong oppression of their boisterous craving for some 'action' during a boring lesson. The heavyweights crush their spirit and extinguish their burning desire to shoot small paper balls at their classmates. This oppression of frisky and high-energy behaviors may be perceived by adult caregivers as a positive outcome of the medications, but the data suggest otherwise [18, Ch. 6]. It is a major adverse outcome that might actually explain why the vast majority of children receiving the medications (77%) are boys [21] (for a further discussion of the gender gap, see Chapter 4).

Proponents of the medications may now ask, "Well, what's wrong with our wish to restrain hyperactive boys through these heavyweight medications?" The answer to this not-so-innocent question is simple. Beside the inherent ethical issue that arises with such an intervention, the apathy, the "asthenia and fatigue", and the "zombie-like demeanor" [2] might gradually develop into "depressed mood" and "diminished interest or pleasure", the two hallmarks of depressive disorders [22, p. 160].

Depression, as implied before, is a common adverse outcome of stimulant medications by itself, alongside multiple other depression-like symptoms, including propensity to cry, sadness, and various sleep-related difficulties (i.e., increased need to sleep, daytime sleepiness, difficulty falling asleep, disturbed sleep, and actual sleep disorder) [2]. This last adverse outcome of sleep dysregulations is even acknowledged by members of the European consensus regarding ADHD [23, p. 24], based on a meta-analysis of nine studies [24]. This is noteworthy, because sleep dysregulations are considered a strong, and even explanatory, risk factor for the onset of depressive disorders [25, 26]. All in all, whether through sleep dysregulations, or through the oppression of high-energy behaviors, empirical evidence suggests that the use of stimulant medications increases the risk for depressive disorders among children [12, 27].

The oppression of the soul

Unfortunately, the behavioral oppression of the previous section is typically accompanied by a strong mental oppression. The relatively scattered cognitive style of the ADHD child is replaced by obsessive thinking patterns, over-focusing, and compulsive behaviors, which could also be interpreted as a positive effect of the medication [18, Ch. 6]. A double-blind study of 45 hyperactive boys treated with ADHD medications (methylphenidate or dextromethamphetamine), conducted by none other than the NIMH itself, revealed that half of the treated children (51%!) developed compulsive behaviors [28]. Indeed, compulsive behaviors may be perceived by teachers or parents as positive outcomes of the medications (e.g., relentless practicing on a musical instrument, over-focusing on school-related work). However, when performed constantly, these behaviors can be redundant and ineffective. Since these compulsory behaviors are sometimes confused with healthy ambitious behaviors, it is important to present the full list here, as formulated by the NIMH researchers. Compulsory behaviors following the use of stimulant medications include: repetitive checking of work; multiple erasures and corrections; pedantry and insistence on negligible details; repeated drawings in the same place; reperforming tasks that seem imperfect; repetitive, purposeless speech or play; and difficulty completing activities at home or at school [28].

Like Obsessive-Compulsive Disorder (OCD), the drug-induced compulsory behaviors may be accompanied by unwanted 'tics' — involuntary motor and/or vocal movements. The NIMH study revealed that 60% (!) of the children using the medications exhibited such tics. In some cases, these tics can cause significant pain. A recent case study article published by physicians who support the use of stimulant medications in ADHD (i.e., they published the case study to help their colleagues enlist patients' medical compliance), describes the case of a 12-year-old girl who bites her tongue and lower lip following a treatment with low doses of methylphenidate [29]. Attempts to switch the methylphenidate with atomoxetine (e.g., Strattera) were unsuccessful, and when the child reverted to using methylphenidate, the bites were so intense and painful that the physicians were forced to discontinue the treatment (I spare the dear reader the unpleasant pictures of the injured tongue and lips presented in the case study). Fortunately, discontinuation of the medication resulted in a cessation of the biting.

The only bright side of the aforementioned case study is probably the fact that the tics were highly noticeable. In many other cases, the tics are more subtle and could be missed by untrained caregivers. Readers should therefore be aware of the list of tics observed in the aforementioned NIMH study. Involuntarily tics in this study included abnormal facial movements, especially around the mouth area (tongue thrusts, licking/smacking/pursing of the tongue, and lateral movements of the chin); stereotypic gestures, such as picking at clothes and fingernails, and repeated rubbing of the chest, eyes, or face; as well as multiple other tics, such as blinking, head jerking, grunting, and involuntary hands or feet trembling [28]. Unfortunately, when these tics are noticed by caregivers and brought to the attention of the physician prescribing the medications, they are sometimes interpreted as signs of an additional psychiatric disorder that should be treated with medications (for a typical escalating dynamic, see Chapter 11).

A method to overpower children

From my perspective, the tics themselves, as well as the other so-called non-serious adverse effects described earlier, are sufficient to compel us to take a break and reconsider if this is how we wish to treat our children, especially considering the invalidity of the disorder (Part One) and the limited efficacy of the medications (Chapters 8 and 9). Yet, from the consensus perspective (which is reluctant to doubt the validity of the disorder or the efficacy of the medications), many physicians prefer to keep experimenting with various brands and doses of stimulant substances, which remain the first-line treatment for ADHD, despite their large collection of adverse events.

For example, a recent study published in 2021 by a research team led by Joseph Biederman (a leading authority in ADHD) found that 41% of adult participants had to switch their prescribed medication, from methylphenidate to amphetamines and vice versa, within a short period of only 3 months, due to poor tolerability [30]. Unfortunately, these alarming findings were not utilized by the researchers to revisit their primary attitude towards stimulant medications, but to call for future research that would help reduce "unnecessary delays" in medication adjustments to patients (p. 310). If they were to ask me (an unrealistic fantasy), I would probably prefer to learn from their findings on adults and ask: Is it really a good idea to administer stimulant medications to children, considering the fact that, even adults who usually take these medications of their own free will, struggle with their adverse outcomes? After all, children are less free to choose whether to use these medications and may be pressured to keep taking them even when they experience negative outcomes [11]. Moreover, children may exhibit lower tolerability than adults. Although not measured directly, medical records of children collected for the COVID-19 study, which was mentioned in Chapter 9, indicated that only about one-quarter of the diagnosed children (24.6%) adhered to their medication plan [31]. Why is it that so few children persist in their pharmacological treatment? The answer is, as shown in my own studies, that despite the alleged consensus (according to which ADHD is said to require daily medical management), most diagnosed children stop taking their medications when they are not in school, mainly because they wish to refrain from experiencing their burdening adverse effects [11, 32].

Psychiatrist Dr. Perter Breggin argues that when young children do use these medications regularly during school hours, they are essentially oppressed by their physicians and adult caregivers (I am sorry, I do not see any other way to phrase this painful position). Children, like the cubs of other mammals, have a natural and healthy desire to run around, investigate, play, and use their senses to explore their environment. The deep engagement in stimulating and playful activities is presumed, from an evolutionary psychology point of view, to promote the development of diverse and flexible responses to startling or unexpected events, such as sudden falls, loss of control, or emotionally-challenging circumstances [33]. When we prescribe them amphetamines, methamphetamines, or methylphenidate, we deprive them of this basic need and cause them to switch off. Studies conducted on monkeys demonstrate that stimulant substances turn the monkey into a submissive animal. Instead of trying to escape from its cage, the monkey hardly moves. It exhibits depressive-like behaviors and useless stereotypic-compulsive behaviors, such as walking in circles or repeatedly chewing its palms [34–36].

Children, like monkeys, may react, more or less the same. Among school children, stimulant medications suppress unwanted classroom behaviors. The child's spark is extinguished. Many treated children no longer seek exciting stimuli in the classroom and are no longer attracted to the window with desperate hopes of discovering something that will save them from the classroom boredom (see also the 'electrifying' study presented in Chapter 5). Instead, they become obsessively focused on school-related tasks, such as copying accurately from the board or completing worksheets meticulously. In this power dynamic between the child and the adult, Breggin argues, the administration of medications serves the one in the powerful position (the adult) who exercises her/his authority over the one in the weak position (the child), thereby turning the child into a submissive, conformist, and obedient child [34]. I would therefore not be surprised if future generations will learn (in futuristic-advanced schools) that, once upon a time, in the early 21st century, pharmacological substances were commonly used as mental chains to oppress and overpower millions of frisky and cheerful children.

Now that we know that the non-serious adverse outcomes of the medications are actually fairly serious and extremely common, we are ready to discuss the documented adverse outcomes that all agree are highly serious. So, buckle your seatbelts and hold on tight as we storm into the next chapter, through the frightening curves of this pharmacological roller-coaster, known as stimulant medications.

References

1. Stanford Children's Health, *ADHD Medication Safe, Experts Say*. Retrieved on November, 2021, Lucile Packard Children's Hospital Stanford. Last retrieved on November 16, 2021 from: https://www.stanfordchildrens.org/en/topic/default?id=adhd-drugs-safe-experts-say-1-3084.
2. Storebø, O.J., *et al.*, *Methylphenidate for attention deficit hyperactivity disorder (ADHD) in children and adolescents–assessment of adverse events in non-randomised studies.* Cochrane Database of Systematic Reviews, 2018. (5).
3. Swanson, J.M., *et al.*, *Young adult outcomes in the follow-up of the multimodal treatment study of attention-deficit/hyperactivity disorder: symptom persistence, source discrepancy, and height suppression.* Journal of Child Psychology and Psychiatry, 2017. **58**(6): p. 663–678.

4. Swanson, J., *et al.*, *Evidence, interpretation, and qualification from multiple reports of long-term outcomes in the Multimodal Treatment Study of Children with ADHD (MTA) Part I: Executive Summary.* Journal of Attention Disorders, 2008. **12**(1): p. 4–14.
5. Charach, A., *et al.*, *Stimulant treatment over 5 years: effects on growth.* Journal of the American Academy of Child & Adolescent Psychiatry, 2006. **45**(4): p. 415–421.
6. Faraone, S.V., *et al.*, *Effect of stimulants on height and weight: a review of the literature.* Journal of the American Academy of Child & Adolescent Psychiatry, 2008. **47**(9): p. 994–1009.
7. Vitiello, B., *Long-Term Effects of Stimulant Medications on the Brain: Possible Relevance to the Treatment of Attention Deficit Hyperactivity Disorder.* Journal of Child and Adolescent Psychopharmacology, 2001. **11**(1): p. 25–34.
8. Aarskog, D., *et al.*, *The effect of the stimulant drugs, dextroamphetamine and methylphenidate, on secretion of growth hormone in hyperactive children.* The Journal of Pediatrics, 1977. **90**(1): p. 136–139.
9. Konrad-Bindl, D.S., U. Gresser, and B.M. Richartz, *Changes in behavior as side effects in methylphenidate treatment: review of the literature.* Neuropsychiatric Disease and Treatment, 2016. **12**: p. 2635.
10. Barkley, R.A., *et al.*, *Side effects of metlyiphenidate in children with attention deficit hyperactivity disorder: a systemic, placebo-controlled evaluation.* Pediatrics, 1990. **86**(2): p. 184–192.
11. Ophir, Y., *Reconsidering the Safety Profile of Stimulant Medications for ADHD.* Ethical Human Psychology and Psychiatry, 2022. **24–1**.
12. Currie, J., M. Stabile, and L. Jones, *Do stimulant medications improve educational and behavioral outcomes for children with ADHD?* Journal of Health Economics, 2014. **37**: p. 58–69.
13. Mayes, S.D., *et al.*, *Methylphenedate and ADHD: Influence of Age, IQ and Neurodevelopmental Status.* Developmental Medicine & Child Neurology, 1994. **36**(12): p. 1099–1107.

14. Swanson, J.M., *et al.*, *Effects of stimulant medication on learning in children with ADHD.* Journal of Learning Disabilities, 1991. **24**(4): p. 219–230.
15. Fiedler, N.L. and D.G. Ullman, *The effects of stimulant drugs on curiosity behaviors of hyperactive boys.* Journal of Abnormal Child Psychology, 1983. **11**(2): p. 193–206.
16. Granger, D.A., C.K. Whalen, and B. Henker, *Perceptions of methylphenidate effects on hyperactive children's peer interactions.* Journal of Abnormal Child Psychology, 1993. **21**(5): p. 535–549.
17. Sax, L., *Boys adrift: The five factors driving the growing epidemic of unmotivated boys and underachieving young men.* 2016: Basic Books.
18. Breggin, P.R., *Psychiatric Drug Withdrawal : A Guide for Prescribers, Therapists, Patients and Their Families.* 2013, New York: Springer Publishing Company.
19. Firestone, P., *et al.*, *Short-term side effects of stimulant medication are increased in preschool children with attention-deficit/hyperactivity disorder: a double-blind placebo-controlled study.* Journal of Child and Adolescent Psychopharmacology, 1998. **8**(1): p. 13–25.
20. Cunningham, C.E. and R.A. Barkley, *The Effects of Methylphenidate on the Mother-child Interactions of Hyperactive Identical Twins.* Developmental Medicine & Child Neurology, 1978. **20**(5): p. 634–642.
21. Fogelman, Y., *et al.*, *Prevalence of and change in the prescription of methylphenidate in Israel over a 2-year period.* CNS Drugs, 2003. **17**(12): p. 915–919.
22. APA, *Diagnostic and Statistical Manual of Mental Disorders (DSM-5®).* 2013: American Psychiatric Association.
23. Kooij, J.J.S., *et al.*, *Updated European Consensus Statement on diagnosis and treatment of adult ADHD.* European Psychiatry, 2019. **56**: p. 14–34.
24. Kidwell, K.M., *et al.*, *Stimulant medications and sleep for youth with ADHD: a meta-analysis.* Pediatrics, 2015. **136**(6): p. 1144–1153.
25. Nutt, D., S. Wilson, and L. Paterson, *Sleep disorders as core symptoms of depression.* Dialogues in Clinical Neuroscience, 2008. **10**(3): p. 329–336.
26. Steiger, A. and M. Pawlowski, *Depression and Sleep.* International Journal of Molecular Sciences, 2019. **20**(3).

27. Cherland, E. and R. Fitzpatrick, *Psychotic side effects of psychostimulants: a 5-year review.* The Canadian Journal of Psychiatry, 1999. **44**(8): p. 811–813.
28. Borcherding, B.G., *et al.*, *Motor/vocal tics and compulsive behaviors on stimulant drugs: is there a common vulnerability?* Psychiatry Research, 1990. **33**(1): p. 83–94.
29. Gokcen, C., M. Karadag, and I. Aksoy, *Methylphenidate Induced Lip and Tongue Biting.* Clinical Psychopharmacology and Neuroscience, 2018. **16**(2): p. 218–220.
30. Biederman, J., *et al.*, *How Frequent Is Switching From an Initial Stimulant Family to the Alternative One in the Clinical Setting?: A Pilot Study of 49 Consecutively Referred Medication-Naive Adults With Attention-Deficit/Hyperactivity Disorder.* Journal of Clinical Psychopharmacology, 2021. **41**(3): p. 310–314.
31. Merzon, E., *et al.*, *ADHD as a Risk Factor for Infection With Covid-19.* Journal of Attention Disorders, 2020. **25**(13): p. 1783–1790.
32. Ophir, Y., *Evidence that the Diagnosis of ADHD Does Not Reflect a Chronic Bio-Medical Disease.* Ethical Human Psychology and Psychiatry, 2022. **23–2**.
33. Spinka, M., R.C. Newberry, and M. Bekoff, *Mammalian play: training for the unexpected.* The Quarterly Review of Biology, 2001. **76**(2): p. 141–168.
34. Breggin, P., *What psychologists and therapists need to know about ADHD and stimulants.* CHANGES-SHEFFIELD-, 2000. **18**(1): p. 13–23.
35. Castner, S.A. and P.S. Goldman-Rakic, *Long-lasting psychotomimetic consequences of repeated low-dose amphetamine exposure in rhesus monkeys.* Neuropsychopharmacology, 1999. **20**(1): p. 10–28.
36. Castner, S.A. and G.V. Williams, *From vice to virtue: Insights from sensitization in the nonhuman primate.* Progress in Neuro-Psychopharmacology and Biological Psychiatry, 2007. **31**(8): p. 1572–1592.

“

“Saying that we’re not sure about the safety and the long-term use of the stimulant medication is nice to say. But the fact is that we know more about the stimulant medications than just about any other medication that’s given to children in medicine... All of the research we have indicates that these drugs are some of the safest that we employ in the field of psychiatry and psychology... we know a lot more than we know about cough medicines and Tylenol and aspirins and other things that children swill whenever they come down with a common cold. Nobody asks those questions about those over-the-counter medications, yet we know substantially less about them.”

Frontline Interview with Russell Barkley. Retrieved in November, 2021 from: PBS (Public Broadcasting Service) [1].

Chapter 11

What are the serious safety concerns of stimulant use?

For those who still believe that the benefits of stimulant medications outweigh their risks, despite their limited efficacy (Chapters 8 and 9) and numerous unwanted adverse effects (Chapter 10), we must continue to discuss the serious and long-term adverse outcomes of the popular medications. Are these powerful and daily used drugs, which cross the blood-brain barrier, really comparable to the very seldom used (especially among children) over-the-counter painkillers, as suggested by Prof. Barkley in the opening quote of this chapter?

In my view, the concerning information provided in the previous chapter is sufficient to answer this question, but skeptic readers might want to know that about 1% of all users of stimulant medications are expected, according to the 2018 Cochrane review (Chapter 10), to suffer from severe outcomes that fall under the unmistakable category of "serious adverse events" [2]. One percent may sound like a relatively small number but given the widespread use of medications for Attention Deficit Hyperactivity Disorder (ADHD) noted in Chapter 7, this figure translates to a very large number of children — a significantly larger estimate than the reported prevalence of these events at the official consumer leaflet [3] presented in Chapter 10 (Figure 3). The current chapter describes four representative serious outcomes of stimulant medications. These include: (1) premature deaths, (2) cardiovascular complications, (3) severe psychiatric conditions, and (4) long-term negative impacts on the brain. Importantly, the last section on brain-related implications also includes an informative discussion of the expected, and highly dangerous adaptation (compensatory) response of the brain, and the grave risk for physiological and psychological addiction to psychoactive substances.

Premature death and suicide

I chose to open the discussion regarding the serious outcomes of the medications with the risk for a premature death, although the absolute risk for premature death during childhood and even adolescence is very low. I would not bother to raise this risk if the proponents of ADHD would not have insisted that the disorder itself is a risk factor for premature death (Chapter 4). But now that they have done so, readers should know that the treatment of choice for ADHD is probably the real factor that increases the risk for premature death, whether through cardiovascular complications (see in the next section) or through the triggering of severe depression (Chapter 10). A major depressive episode is often accompanied by painful thoughts about death and suicide [4] and suicide rates are ever increasing in the US, since about 2005-2007 [5], especially among adolescent boys [6] who are, as we already know from Chapters 2 and 4, at greater risk to be diagnosed with ADHD.

Beginning in 2007, suicide rates among male youths increased by an annual percentage change of about 3.4%, with a sharp increase in 2015 of about 13.6% [6]. There could be, of course, multiple reasons for this increase, including for example, the emergence of smartphones and other screen technologies [7], but these reasons are yet to be proven [8], while the dramatic increase in stimulant use, which occurred more or less in the same period, cannot be ruled out as a plausible risk factor. A recent study found that amphetamine use for ADHD increased 2.5-fold from 2006 to 2016 [9]. Specifically, methylphenidate use peaked in 2012, and the growing use of amphetamines overtook its place in 2016.

I am the last person to argue that the aforementioned trends are sufficient to conclude that stimulant use is related, in a direct relationship, to suicide attempts. However, I would not dismiss this hypothesis. A large study of the UK general practice research database revealed that the risk for actual suicide deaths is significantly increased among adolescents and young adults who used stimulant medications (*Standardized Mortality Ratio* = 1.84), compared to non-users [10]. For younger treated children, aged 11-14, the absolute risk in this study was, of course, much smaller, but when a comparison was made with a cohort of unmedicated children, the relative risk for suicide death among the medicated children was enormous (Standardized Mortality Ratio = 161.91).

Oddly, despite these warning signs, the risk for suicide is not mentioned explicitly as a potential adverse outcome in the consumer leaflet presented in the previous chapter (Figure 3, Chapter 10). The item "thoughts or attempts of suicide (including completed suicide)" only appears in a separate section that lists "additional side-effects that occurred with other medications that contain the same active ingredient". This "additional" list comprises 15 bullet points, each describing one or more adverse outcomes. The critical risk for suicide is buried (I am sorry there is no better word to describe this concealment practice) in the third and the longest bullet point, which comprises no less than 16, not necessarily related adverse outcomes, such as excessive awareness of surroundings, feeling unusually excited, change in sex drive, and confusion. This sense of concealment contrasts the findings from my own study, in which 3.2% of the participants reported that the medications for ADHD triggered unwanted suicidal thoughts [3].

Cardiovascular complications

Another path to premature death may be through the negative effects of the stimulant substances on the cardiovascular system. We know from studies on adults and on the elderly, for example, that the initiation of methylphenidate increases the risk of dangerous cardiovascular events and even sudden deaths [11–13]. Indeed, the literature on cardiovascular complications following the administration of stimulant medications is somewhat mixed, but the warning signs, especially in childhood, cannot be ignored.

Gould and colleagues [14] for example, detected 564 cases of sudden deaths of children and adolescents (aged 7–19) that occurred in the US between the years 1985–1996. They tracked the various factors that could have contributed to the occurrence of these deaths, by comparing the sample of sudden deaths with a parallel sample of children killed in car accidents and found that the risk of unexplained sudden death increased dramatically when the child was using stimulant medications ($OR = 7.4$). Of course, we have no way to determine the precise cause of this observed increased risk. However, the researchers proposed that the increased risk for sudden death results from the negative effects of the stimulants on the cardiovascular system [14]. This hypothesis does not appear out of nowhere. Even the most ardent supporters of the medications recognize the risk for cardiovascular problems following the use of stimulant medications [15]. This known risk may explain why the Lancet Child & Adolescent Health Journal has issued recently special guidelines for starting stimulant medications during the COVID-19 pandemic [16]. According to the new guidelines, physicians should avoid initiating new, stimulant-based treatments during the COVID-19 pandemic, to individuals who have a medical history of breathing or heart problems or those who have a family history of early (<40 years) sudden deaths.

Although not mentioned explicitly, I suspect that the studies on ADHD and COVID-19 mentioned in Chapter 4 [17, 18] hide a troubling piece of information regarding a potential serious risk of the medications. Briefly, two publications in the *Journal of Attention Disorders*, by Merzon and colleagues posited that ADHD is a risk factor for COVID-19 — a study from 2020 reported of an increased risk for COVID-19 *infections* [17] and a study from 2021 reported of an increased risk for *severity* of COVID-related outcomes, that is: symptoms and hospitalizations [18].

Notably, both studies relied on similar datasets from the large Israeli health service of 'Leumit'. The 2020 dataset included all the service members who were tested for COVID-19 during a period of *3 months* (February 1 — April 30, 2020) and the 2021 dataset included all the members (aged 5-60 years) who were tested *positive* for COVID-19, during an overlapping period of *5 months* (February 1 — June 30, 2020). Aside from the multiple biases detected in the 2020 study (see Chapter 12), the similarity between the two datasets produced several discrepancies, which challenge the conclusions of the two studies [19]. For example, in contrast to the 2020 study, which stratified the ADHD cases to treated and untreated individuals (a methodological operation that was utilized by the authors to argue, as mentioned in Chapter 9, that the medications are needed to mitigate the risk for COVID-19 infections), the 2021 study does not provide this information. This last omission is particularly surprising considering the corresponding author's statement in a TV interview (in Hebrew) that the **main headline** from her 2020 study should be that people with ADHD can take medications and reduce their risk to catch the virus (a saved copy of this TV interview is available by Y.O.). Together, the fact that the 2020 study reporting of medications does not report of severe COVID outcomes (Chapter 4) and the fact that the 2021 study reporting of severe COVID outcomes does not report of medication use, do not allow us to rule out the possibility that stimulant medications constitute an artifact that could explain the observed link between ADHD and severity of COVID-19 outcomes [19].

We should therefore ask ourselves, what is more theoretically reasonable, that the severe reactions to a respiratory virus are a product of ADHD (a condition characterized by unrelated behaviors, such as hyperactivity or distractibility) or of a regular use of psychoactive drugs that impact cardiovascular functions? In fact, even Merzon and colleagues do not seem to speculate that the very existence of ADHD, by itself, can contribute to the increased risk for COVID-related outcomes. In their introductory justification for their 2021 study, they hypothesized that the link between ADHD and severe COVID-19 outcomes would be evident, "even if only by association with other clinical correlates" [18, p. 492]. These hypothesized mediating/moderating "clinical correlates" are, according to the introductory justification of the study, conditions that seem much more related to COVID-19 outcomes, such as: obesity, asthma, and smoking.

Interestingly however, the authors do not conduct a mediation analysis or a moderation analysis to support their implied hypothesis (e.g., the provided regression analysis does not include interaction effects). On the contrary, they conducted a logistic regression analysis that produced unique effects for each of the examined variables. In other words, they practically controlled for the "clinical correlates" that were proposed in their introductory justification and presented an analysis that showed that ADHD is associated with severe outcomes of COVID-19, above and beyond these correlates [19]. Moreover, the "clinical correlates" proposed in the introduction — the asthma, the obesity, and the smoking — did not contribute to the unified prediction model of severe COVID-19 outcomes (i.e., their *Adjusted Odds Ratios* were **not** significant). These non-findings are particularly strange in light of what we know about the risks for COVID-19 outcomes [e.g., 20, 21, 22].

I therefore strongly recommend considering the alternative hypothesis that was eliminated in this study, that is, the hypothesis regarding the potentially dangerous impact of the medications on COVID-related outcomes. Generally,

I avoid mentioning studies in a 'grocery list' fashion, but in light of the close link between cardiovascular disease and severe COVID-19 outcomes, including COVID-related mortalities [20, 23], it is important that we internalize the robust evidence regarding the cardiovascular risks of the medications, as all stimulants have US Food and Drug Administration (FDA) warnings on their consumer leaflets regarding potential cardiovascular implications [24].

The large Australian Raine Study mentioned in Chapter 9, for example, suspected that stimulant medications cause a significant increase in the user's diastolic blood pressure over time [25]. Similar warnings appeared in a Canadian study. A study that investigated 2,013 middle-school children (5th to 8th graders) in southern Ontario documented an increase in systolic and diastolic blood pressure alongside a significant increase in heart rate among medicated children [26]. Notably, the levels of heart rate and blood pressure among diagnosed children who were not using the medications were equivalent to the levels among non-diagnosed children. Complementing this picture, a wide-scope retrospective study from Florida on 55,383 children and adolescents with ADHD found that the use of stimulants was associated with increased risk for cardiac emergency department visits [27]. Here too, diagnosed children who did not use stimulant medications had the same (very low) risk for emergency room visits as the non-diagnosed population. Finally, a prospective longitudinal study that investigated all the children born in Denmark over the course of an entire decade found that stimulant medications **doubled the risk** of developing cardiac events [28].

Indeed, without sufficient longitudinal Randomized Controlled Trials (RCTs), we cannot draw conclusive conclusions regarding direct causal relationships. However, we cannot ignore the clear writing on the (heart) wall either. The accumulating evidence from the past decades, as reported in a recent literature review published in the well-acknowledged *Journal of the American College of Cardiology*, suggests that ADHD medications can cause dysregulations in resting heart rate and blood pressure, and that there is a serious risk that prolonged use of these medications would eventually lead to decreased heart functions (non-ischemic cardiomyopathy), "broken heart syndrome" (Takotsubo cardiomyopathy), and even sudden deaths [24]. It is now clear why all stimulants have FDA warnings regarding cardiac risks, as mentioned earlier, and why the Israeli package insert (leaflet) instructs patients to inform their physicians (before they start taking the medication) about any "heart defects", "heart problems", or "medical history of sudden death or irregular heart rate" in their family (Figure 3, Chapter 10).

Severe psychiatric reactions — psychosis and mania

One of the justifications made for treating young children with powerful stimulant substances, which are known to have cardiac risks, is that these medications are necessary to reduce the risk for future, and more serious, psychiatric conditions such as psychotic or manic episodes [29]. The data, however, indicate the exact opposite. Over a decade ago, researchers from the FDA conducted a thorough review of 49 RCTs performed by the drug manufacturers themselves (who, of course, seek to demonstrate the efficacy and safety of their medications). This investigation revealed concerning abnormal rates of psychotic and manic expressions among the participating children in the intervention arms of these RCTs. These included visual and sensory hallucinations, which involved the (imaginary) appearance of insects, snakes, and worms [30].

Corroborating with the FDA findings, a large study conducted in Taiwan on 73,049 children and adolescents with ADHD — a study that actually tried to prove the dangerous aspects of ADHD by linking it to future psychotic disorders — found that diagnosed children who were treated with methylphenidate were at a significantly greater risk for developing a psychotic disorder compared to diagnosed children who did not use medications [31]. Similarly, a study that focused on adolescents with bipolar disorder, found that the onset of this severe psychiatric condition was earlier (in age) among adolescents who used stimulant medications, compared to adolescents who did not use these medications [32].

Regrettably, empirical findings in this field are not always presented in a transparent and objective manner (Chapter 12). A recent large study from Sweden for example, concluded that "contrary to clinical concerns", there is "no evidence that initiation of methylphenidate treatment increases the risk of psychotic events in adolescents and young adults" [33, p. 651]. However, when I dived into its methodology, I was stunned to find that the researchers disregarded most of their dataset. Of the 61,814 participants who used the medications, the researchers decided to analyze data from only 23,898 participants (38.7%). Their reasons for excluding so many participants were: deaths (0.6%), additional use of medication other than methylphenidate (11.2%), and most oddly, "inappropriate age" (49.5%) (page 654). About half of the dataset, which comprised thousands of children who started their methylphenidate treatment before the age of 12, was completely ignored. Why would scientists engage in such a bold misrepresentation of their data? Chapter 12 tries to answer this (in my opinion, horrifying) question, but let us just mention here that four of the authors of this study reported of relationships with pharmaceutical companies. This does not necessarily mean that the researchers were fully aware of this scientific misconduct, but, together with the intensity of the observed bias, these conflicts of interest undermine the *internal validity* of the conclusions of the study.

In stark contrast to the misrepresented Swedish study, a time-worn longitudinal study from Canada which followed 192 diagnosed children for five years revealed that almost **10%** of the children who were treated with stimulants (primarily methylphenidate) developed psychotic symptoms. Of this group, 88% exhibited the symptoms **before** the age of 12 [34]. This finding has two implications to our discussion here. First, according to this study, the serious risk for psychosis is by no means a rare risk, as one might think. Second, the appearance of the psychotic symptoms before the age of 12 suggests that the aforementioned decision to disregard thousands of treated children, in the Swedish study, might not have been so innocent. One can only imagine what the real risk for a psychosis reaction in this study was, before the blatant manipulation of the data.

Psychosis is not the only severe psychiatric reaction that could be triggered by stimulant use. The aforementioned longitudinal Canadian study found that about 12% of the treated children developed symptoms of mood disorders (a cluster of disorders from the previous edition of the *Diagnostic and Statistical Manual of Mental Disorders* (*DSM*), which included unipolar (depressive) and bipolar (manic-depressive) disorders [34]. Overall, at least 18% of the treated children in this study developed one or more severe psychiatric condition — a huge number by all accounts, which suggests that serious adverse outcomes are, in fact, pretty common.

Peeling off poor scientific bandages

Take note of what happened next in this study on severe psychiatric reactions [34]. Following the onset of the new psychiatric symptoms, some of the children were clinically labeled with an additional psychiatric diagnosis, pervasive developmental disorder, or bipolar disorder, which is typically treated with other pharmacological substances (e.g., antidepressants, mood stabilizers), sometimes in addition to the stimulant medications already in use. In such cases, proponents of the pharmacological treatment tend to claim that the severe mental illness existed, in some latent form, before the initiation of the stimulant treatment. Sometimes they even argue that children who are given the medications for long periods are usually the ones who suffer the most severe ADHD symptoms, and that these severe symptoms are actually indicative of their prodrome severe psychiatric state. From their perspective, the vulnerable child was 'lucky' to receive the stimulant treatment, because it helped to attenuate early expressions of his/her severe illness, and perhaps even to delay its full-blown clinical onset. However, this non-parsimonious justification is a poor scientific bandage, as more than half of all psychotic outbreaks in the Canadian study occurred in close proximity to the beginning of the stimulant treatment, right after the first dose, or within a few weeks after the initiation of the treatment [34]. In other words, this study provided strong indications for a direct, causal link between stimulant use and psychiatric reactions.

Additional support for this direct link between stimulant use and severe psychiatric reactions appears in a more recent, and much larger, study of 12,856 young adults [35]. This study revealed an increased risk of hospitalization for psychosis or mania within 60 days from the first administration of the stimulants (*OR* = 1.86). Moreover, 45% of the people who were discharged from the hospital with a prescription for stimulant medications had to be hospitalized again shortly after they were discharged, because the psychotic or manic episodes returned. These findings are consistent with previous findings from animal studies, in which monkeys demonstrated stereotypic gestures and hallucination-like behaviors following the administration of low doses of stimulant substances [36, 37]. Now, judge for yourself which came first, the onset of the severe psychiatric reaction or the initiation of the treatment of choice for ADHD?

Unfortunately, scientific findings that challenge the safety of ADHD medications, such as the ones described in this chapter, tend to be silenced quickly by parties of interest (Chapter 12), and many physicians who prescribe these medications are left oblivious to their risks. Yet, there are some physicians who have emerged from the silence and dared to publish dreadful case studies on the serious adverse outcomes of ADHD medications.

The case of Billy

As early as 1967, years before the introduction of the contemporary formulation of ADHD (Chapter 3), the *Canadian Medical Association Journal* published a case study of amphetamine-induced psychosis [38]. Billy (a pseudonym), an 8-year-old boy with a perfectly normal developmental medical history, was diagnosed by a private psychiatrist with brain damage (see the introduction for the various incarnations of ADHD), due to his poor academic performance and poor behavior in the classroom. To manage this (neurobiological) problem, the psychiatrist recommended that Billy will start taking prescribed amphetamines.

One day, shortly after Christmas, Billy began to hallucinate that unidentified figures were throwing snowballs at him, spying on him, and talking about him. He heard strange noises (which he demonstrated to his parents by pinching his nose), which did not allow him to fall asleep. He also felt that someone was touching his thighs and genitals, and no one could convince him that these experiences were not real. One time, out of panic, he jumped off a trampoline in a dangerous manner, because he thought someone was looking at him from around the corner.

Billy was in an endless medical loop. When he tried to stop the stimulant treatment, the hallucinations stopped but his hyperactivity increased, and he was expelled from school. When he resumed taking the medication (so that he could go back to school), his paranoid delusions and hallucinations returned [38]. This early case study supports the conclusions from the previous empirical discussion regarding the potential causal link between stimulant use and psychotic expressions among some children. The hallucinations and delusions appeared when Billy used the stimulant medication and disappeared when he stopped using it.

The case of Oliver

A more recent case study published in the prestigious *American Journal of Psychiatry* relates the story of Oliver (a pseudonym), a young boy who had attention difficulties [39]. At the age of 7, Oliver began using the popular medication of methylphenidate and, apart from "mild anorexia", everyone in his surroundings were satisfied with the improvement in his ADHD symptoms. Suddenly, at 8 years old, without any prior, personal or familial psychiatric history, and shortly after recovering from a seasonal flu, Oliver suddenly developed visual and auditory hallucinations. He saw old people who were not there and felt a strong need to throw himself down the stairs. Oliver felt constant fear and anxiety. He cried a lot at school and was unwilling to leave his mother's side. Fortunately, lowering the dose of the medication alleviated Oliver's psychotic symptoms and the discontinuation of the medication eliminated them altogether [39].

The case of Elijah

Last, but not easy to read, is the case of Elijah (a pseudonym). Changes in the dose of methylphenidate (in this case, Concerta) given to this ten-year-old boy diagnosed with ADHD caused severe sensory hallucinations [40]. Elijah felt that there was fluid dripping down his legs due to a genital injury (that had not occurred in reality). Elijah believed that his glans penis and scrotum were damaged in such a way that his urine seeped down towards his feet. These hallucinations were accompanied by burning sensations in these body areas and a feeling as if he had a stone in the tip of his penis. In addition, he experienced sensory hallucinations in which he felt insects crawling under his skin and inside his hair and mouth. As a result, he developed cleansing motions and rituals to remove them. Due to these symptoms, the methylphenidate treatment was stopped and **within two days**, the entire psychotic manifestation disappeared, including multiple other somatic sensations [40].

I apologize to the readers for bringing forth such unpleasant case descriptions. However, these graphic descriptions are highly needed in the face of the silencing practices that are prevalent in the field (Chapter 12). Indeed, case studies may be anecdotal, and we should be careful not to over-generalize their conclusions. However, there is abundant evidence, as mentioned above, from both human and nonhuman primate studies that repeated exposure to stimulant substances, such as amphetamines, can trigger psychosis-like behaviors [e.g., 30-32, 36, 37]. Some of these severe psychiatric reactions may pass, once the treatment is terminated, as demonstrated in the case studies above but, in some cases of prolonged use of stimulant medications, the impact on the brain could be permanent and devastating, as will be illustrated next.

Long-term impacts on the brain (including addiction)

We are used to being told that the "brain disorder" of ADHD involves serious negative implications (Introduction). However, when we dive into the empirical studies that are said to support this claim, we sometimes discover that they 'forgot' to compare these negative implications between treated and untreated individuals (Chapter 4). Without this comparison, we cannot determine whether the brain-related implications arise from the disorder, or from the treatment. When such comparisons are conducted, disturbing findings are sometimes exposed.

A recent study for example, which reported of a 2.4-fold increased risk for a brain disease of the basal ganglia and cerebellum areas among a gross sample of 31,769 adults with ADHD, revealed that the risk was particularly increased, at **8.6-fold**, among the subgroup of 4,960 adults who were using medications for their ADHD [41]. The increased risk in the remaining sample, for whom information about medication use was **not** available (i.e., this group included both treated and untreated individuals), was only 1.8-fold. Not surprisingly, like in the previous section, non-parsimonious rationalizations were proposed in this study as well. The authors of this study speculated that treated individuals were at greater risk because their ADHD was more severe in the first place (compared with the untreated individuals). But is this the most reasonable explanation for the observed results? The answer to this question is provided below, in the form of a detailed discussion of the expected implications of prolonged use of stimulants on the human brain, including the brain's anticipated, and highly dangerous, adaptation response, which underlies the risk for substance use disorders and other addictive behaviors.

The real "brain deficit" and "chemical imbalance"

Readers so far probably remember from the Introduction and from Chapter 6 that consensual figures in the field typically refer to ADHD as an objective brain deficit that causes biochemical dysregulations of key neurotransmitters, such as dopamine and norepinephrine [42]. Although this latter, "chemical imbalance" hypothesis was refuted in Chapter 6 and denounced by mainstream psychiatrists [43], the desirable benefits of stimulants are still attributed to the blockage of the (presumably dysregulated) reuptake process of these neurotransmitters [44]. Through this blockage, as well as through artificial induction of additional levels of dopamine or norepinephrine [42], increased levels of neurotransmitters remain in the synapse for longer periods, thus allowing the individual to realize their full cognitive potential (Chapter 6).

Now, for the purposes of this discussion, let's assume that there is some degree of truth in the chemical imbalance hypothesis, and that children with

ADHD are in a constant state of insufficient levels of neurotransmitters; how then will the medications 'fix' this problem? Even if medications are able to fill the presumed neurotransmitter gap in the short term, what will happen to the child's brain in the long term? How would the brain react to a recurrent administration of artificial neurotransmitter enhancer? Considering the lack of high-quality longitudinal studies in humans (Chapter 9), and the understandable ethical limitations that are involved in such studies, in order to answer these questions, we must turn to animal studies, which allow researchers a greater latitude in analyzing the long-term effects of stimulant medications on the animal's brain.

There is substantial evidence that recurrent administration of high doses of stimulant substances to animals is toxic [45], but even low doses that resemble clinical doses in ADHD can cause long-term changes in the animal's brain [46]. A review of non-human primate studies, for example, revealed that repeated exposure to low doses of amphetamine can lead to long-term brain deficits [47]. This brain deficit is manifested in a reduced synaptic plasticity (the brain's way to adapt to changing circumstances) and a growing degeneration of neurons in the prefrontal cortex and the striatum [48] — the same principal regions that are hypothesized to be impaired in ADHD.

Repeated exposure to stimulants in primates also impairs their executive functions [47] — the same cognitive abilities that are presumed to be impaired in ADHD. Studies on mice and rats have yielded similar results. Chronic 'treatment' with methylphenidate increased impulsive-like behaviors, and triggered oxidative stress and inflammation of brain cells, which ultimately damaged DNA molecules [49], leading to a corruption of neurons, both in the cortex and in deeper regions of the brain [50, 51].

Not only has ADHD never been proven to be a "brain disorder" of a "chemical imbalance" (Part One), the animal studies reviewed here suggest that there is also ample evidence that the treatment of choice for ADHD can trigger biochemical dysregulations and create a sort of a brain disorder. In fact, the extensive brain deficits triggered by stimulant use seem to originate from exactly the same brain processes that were intended to be improved through the use of these medications. In one of the first studies that investigated the long-term effects of methylphenidate in mice, the researchers observed a significant reduction in the density of dopamine transporters in the striatum — a persistent reduction that lasted even after the discontinuation of the medication [52]. Another study found that methylphenidate elicited a chain of inflammatory-defensive responses in the brain. The researchers observed an increase in microglial cells (i.e., the cells that are designed to protect the central nervous system) located at the basal ganglia region, as well as a decrease in the number of dopamine-secreting cells in the striatum, within the substantia nigra pars compacta [53].

The reason I mention these specific regions by name is that these very regions are known to play a critical role in basic reinforcement processes [54]. In fact, there is a growing body of evidence that prolonged use of stimulants has a direct impact on the motivation and reward centers of the brain [55]. The repeated administration of the stimulant substance disrupts the dopaminergic system [56], reduces the mouse's sensitivity to reinforcements, and depresses its overall behavior [57]. Like children (Chapter 10), mice that are exposed to methylphenidate become apathetic. They are less responsive to typical reinforcements (e.g., sugar), new and intriguing stimuli, and sexual activities [58]. The mice become reluctant to spontaneously explore their environment the way they used to do in the past, and they appear to external viewers as 'depressed' animals [59]. Like addicts, the only thing that might comfort the mice now is another dose of the drug (see next).

Physiological and psychological addictions

"As with all stimulants," the official Israeli consumer leaflet of Ritalin brought in Chapter 10 states, "**this medicine can be addictive and abused by certain people**" (bold in the original text). Not only do the stimulants inflict direct adverse effects as documented above, they also trigger a series of indirect adverse outcomes, such as addictive behaviors, mainly as the result of the brain's natural attempts to cope with the externally induced drug (which is essentially identified by the brain as a neurotoxin that should be eliminated). Indeed, the leaflet immediately continues to calm the consumer of the drug by predicting, in a clear-cut manner that: "If you take it [the Ritalin] properly, as instructed by the doctor, abuse or dependence should not occur, neither now nor in the future." However, the available evidence does not seem to support this decisive statement. After all, we barely have high-quality longitudinal controlled experiments (Chapter 9).

In contrast to the (false) reassuring message of the leaflet, there is substantial evidence today that prolonged usage of stimulants, even in careful, medically controlled doses, can lead to further addictive behaviors and substance use disorders [60]. Prof. Nadine Lambert, as you might remember from the Introduction, presented such evidence in the founding Consensus Development Conference. Results from her prospective longitudinal study suggested that the use of ADHD medications in childhood might lead to increased smoking and drug abuse (mainly cocaine) in adulthood [61].

The risk for further problematic drug abuse may originate from psychological factors (see further in this chapter), as well as from pure biological adaptation reactions to the externally induced drug. Consider, for example, the findings from the doctoral dissertation of Emanual Quansah from the Center for Neurodegenerative Science at the Van Andel Research Institute. Through a variety of bioanalytical methods, Quansah compared the brains of mice that received methylphenidate for a short period of time with the brains of mice that received the medication for a long period of time. This comparison revealed that the prolonged exposure to methylphenidate caused multiple long-term biochemical changes in the animals' brain [62]. In particular, long-termed treated mice exhibited a significant increase in dopamine transporters [63] — the very proteins that are supposed to remove the excess dopamine from the synapse in the reuptake process (Chapter 6). It seems that the animal's brain realizes that it is under a dopamine 'attack' and consequently produces more and more transporters to eliminate the excess dopamine.

It is now easy to understand (1) why the desired effects of the medication weaken over time, (2) why there is an exacerbation of ADHD-like symptoms after prolonged usage of the medication, and (3) why, when an attempt is made to stop the medication, there is an increase in ADHD symptoms, as well as other, severe withdrawal symptoms [64]. Even if stimulant medications appear to be effective to some extent in the short term, after a while, they can cause long-term changes in the dopaminergic system. These changes constitute the physiological basis of drug dependency and addictive behaviors, phenomena well known to us from people who abuse stimulant substances regularly [65]. They also explain why hyperactive mice (yes, there are such creatures) that were given methylphenidate were later more vulnerable to cocaine use (when offered to them), compared with a control sample of mice that were not given methylphenidate [66]. In other words, 'soft' stimulant use can cause further physiological addiction to more dangerous 'hard-core' psychoactive substances.

It is difficult to scrutinize pure physiological addiction (that originates from biochemical changes in the dopaminergic system) from the more subjective psychological feeling of addiction that is based on behavioral conditioning, as well as on other (somewhat more amorphic) psychological factors, such as learned helplessness or poor self-esteem. However, it is reasonable to argue that daily medication use may also produce a subjective sense of dependence. A recent Israeli longitudinal study on 6,830 children and adolescents, published in a consensual psychiatric journal (*European Child & Adolescent Psychiatry*), reported that prolonged use of ADHD medication in childhood predicted future use of antidepressant medications in adolescence [67]. Children who adhered to their medication plan of methylphenidate in childhood had a 50% higher chance of using antidepressants in adolescence, compared to children who did not adhere to their medication plan.

To explain these disturbing results, the researchers posited that the increased risk for antidepressant use was more pronounced among the children who used methylphenidate regularly, because their ADHD was more severe in the first place. Like the aforementioned rationalizations of the previous sections, the label of ADHD here was presumed to disguise more severe psychiatric conditions (in this case, depression). However, when considering the findings from the animal studies presented here, the studies presented in the previous section on severe psychiatric reactions, and the studies on depression from Chapter 10, it seems to me that this explanation is unjustified and not scientifically parsimonious (see also the General Discussion).

In my opinion, there are more plausible and more parsimonious explanations, which do not exclude one another, according to which: (1) stimulant medications inhibit spontaneous and curious behaviors and increase depression-like symptoms and behaviors (Chapter 10); (2) overloading of externally induced substances on the central nervous system activates compensatory brain mechanisms, which could lead to physiological addiction; and (3) relying on medications for academic/behavioral success (like on scaffolding) at a young age instills in the child a psychological perception that life problems and challenges can, or should be, solved with pills. When the going gets tough, the tough get Ritalin; when it gets tougher, the tough get Prozac or Clonex or Risperdal or Lithium — big solutions in small pills, available by your local family doctor.

Medication safety in a nutshell

Prof. Barkley is probably right. "We know more about the stimulant medications than just about any other medication that's given to children in medicine", as stated in the opening quote of this chapter [1]. Here is a brief 'elevator speech' description of what we know of stimulant medications: Long-standing solutions never come in magic pills (Chapter 9). Not only are the medications not effective in the long run, they are also quite dangerous. They have numerous 'non-serious' side effects, which are essentially pretty averse experiences (Chapter 10), and they can create severe long-term physical and psychological damage (the current chapter). A constant use of stimulant medications for ADHD is, by no means, equivalent to the rare use of "Tylenol and aspirins". If anything, daily usage of such dangerous and addictive substances should be compared to the use of related illicit stimulant substances, such as cocaine and other amphetamines [68] that are known to trigger the adverse outcomes described in this chapter:

the cardiovascular dysregulations, the psychotic reactions, and the suicide ideation [69].

And yet, Barkley's beliefs regarding the safety of the medications, from the opening quote of this chapter, are widely common among clinicians and patients. How is it possible that so many people believe that stimulant medications are "the safest that we employ", despite the massive evidence that they are not safe at all? To answer this question, we ought to take a close look, in the next chapter, at the powerful forces that fuel the silencing practices within the scientific discourse on ADHD and stimulant medications.

References

1. Frontline Interview with Russell Barkley, *Interview Russell Barkley*. Retrieved on November 2021, Frontline | PBS (Public Broadcasting Service). Last Retrieved on November 16, 2021 from: https://www.pbs.org/wgbh/pages/frontline/shows/medicating/interviews/barkley.html.
2. Storebø, O.J., *et al.*, *Methylphenidate for attention deficit hyperactivity disorder (ADHD) in children and adolescents–assessment of adverse events in non-randomised studies.* Cochrane Database of Systematic Reviews, 2018(5).
3. Ophir, Y., *Reconsidering the Safety Profile of Stimulant Medications for ADHD.* Ethical Human Psychology and Psychiatry, 2022. **24–1**.
4. APA, *Diagnostic and Statistical Manual of Mental Disorders (DSM-5®).* 2013: American Psychiatric Association.
5. Rossen, L.M., *et al.*, *County-level trends in suicide rates in the US, 2005–2015.* American Journal of Preventive Medicine, 2018. **55**(1): p. 72–79.
6. Mishara, B.L. and S. Stijelja, *Trends in US Suicide Deaths, 1999 to 2017, in the Context of Suicide Prevention Legislation.* JAMA Pediatrics, 2020. **174**(5): p. 499–500.
7. Twenge, J.M., *et al.*, *Increases in Depressive Symptoms, Suicide-Related Outcomes, and Suicide Rates Among U.S. Adolescents After 2010 and Links to Increased New Media Screen Time.* Clinical Psychological Science, 2017. **6**(1): p. 3–17.

8. Ophir, Y., Y. Lipshits-Braziler, and H. Rosenberg, *New-Media Screen Time is Not (Necessarily) Linked to Depression: Comments on Twenge, Joiner, Rogers, and Martin (2018).* Clinical Psychological Science, 2019: p. 2167702619849412.
9. Piper, B.J., *et al.*, *Trends in use of prescription stimulants in the United States and Territories, 2006 to 2016.* PloS one, 2018. **13**(11): p. e0206100.
10. McCarthy, S., *et al.*, *Mortality associated with attention-deficit hyperactivity disorder (ADHD) drug treatment.* Drug Safety, 2009. **32**(11): p. 1089–1096.
11. Tadrous, M., *et al.*, *Assessment of Stimulant Use and Cardiovascular Event Risks Among Older Adults.* JAMA Network Open, 2021. **4**(10): p. e2130795-e2130795.
12. Schelleman, H., *et al.*, *Methylphenidate and Risk of Serious Cardiovascular Events in Adults.* American Journal of Psychiatry, 2012. **169**(2): p. 178–185.
13. Mosholder, A.D., *et al.*, *Incidence of Heart Failure and Cardiomyopathy Following Initiation of Medications for Attention-Deficit/Hyperactivity Disorder: A Descriptive Study.* Journal of Clinical Psychopharmacology, 2018. **38**(5).
14. Gould, M.S., *et al.*, *Sudden Death and Use of Stimulant Medications in Youths.* American Journal of Psychiatry, 2009. **166**(9): p. 992–1001.
15. Faraone, S.V., *The pharmacology of amphetamine and methylphenidate: Relevance to the neurobiology of attention-deficit/hyperactivity disorder and other psychiatric comorbidities.* Neuroscience & Biobehavioral Reviews, 2018. **87**: p. 255–270.
16. Cortese, S., *et al.*, *Starting ADHD medications during the COVID-19 pandemic: recommendations from the European ADHD Guidelines Group.* The Lancet Child & Adolescent Health, 2020. **4**(6): p. e15.
17. Merzon, E., *et al.*, *ADHD as a Risk Factor for Infection With Covid-19.* Journal of Attention Disorders, 2020. **25**(13): p. 1783–1790.
18. Merzon, E., *et al.*, *The Association between ADHD and the Severity of COVID-19 Infection.* Journal of Attention Disorders, 2021. **26**(4): p. 491–501.
19. Ophir, Y. and Y. Shir-Raz, *Discrepancies in Studies on ADHD and COVID-19 Raise Concerns Regarding the Risks of Stimulant Treatments During an Active Pandemic.* Accepted Manuscript. Ethical Human Psychology and Psychiatry.
20. Williamson, E.J., *et al.*, *Factors associated with COVID-19-related death using OpenSAFELY.* Nature, 2020. **584**(7821): p. 430–436.

21. Rivera-Izquierdo, M., *et al.*, *Sociodemographic, clinical and laboratory factors on admission associated with COVID-19 mortality in hospitalized patients: A retrospective observational study.* PloS one, 2020. **15**(6): p. e0235107.
22. Reddy, R.K., *et al.*, *The effect of smoking on COVID-19 severity: A systematic review and meta-analysis.* Journal of Medical Virology, 2021. **93**(2): p. 1045–1056.
23. Clerkin, K.J., *et al.*, *COVID-19 and cardiovascular disease.* Circulation, 2020. **141**(20): p. 1648–1655.
24. Torres-Acosta, N., *et al.*, *Cardiovascular Effects of ADHD Therapies.* Journal of the American College of Cardiology, 2020. **76**(7): p. 858–866.
25. Whitely, M., *The rise and fall of ADHD child prescribing in Western Australia: Lessons and implications.* Australian & New Zealand Journal of Psychiatry, 2012. **46**(5): p. 400–403.
26. Amour, M.D.S., *et al.*, *What is the effect of ADHD stimulant medication on heart rate and blood pressure in a community sample of children?* Canadian Journal of Public Health, 2018. **109**(3): p. 395–400.
27. Winterstein, A.G., *et al.*, *Cardiac safety of central nervous system stimulants in children and adolescents with attention-deficit/hyperactivity disorder.* Pediatrics, 2007. **120**(6): p. e1494-e1501.
28. Dalsgaard, S., *et al.*, *Cardiovascular safety of stimulants in children with attention-deficit/hyperactivity disorder: a nationwide prospective cohort study.* Journal of Child and Adolescent Psychopharmacology, 2014. **24**(6): p. 302–310.
29. Biederman, J., *et al.*, *Do Stimulants Protect Against Psychiatric Disorders in Youth With ADHD? A 10-Year Follow-up Study.* Pediatrics, 2009. **124**(1): p. 71.
30. Mosholder, A.D., *et al.*, *Hallucinations and other psychotic symptoms associated with the use of attention-deficit/hyperactivity disorder drugs in children.* Pediatrics, 2009. **123**(2): p. 611–616.
31. Shyu, Y.-C., *et al.*, *Attention-deficit/hyperactivity disorder, methylphenidate use and the risk of developing schizophrenia spectrum disorders: A nationwide population-based study in Taiwan.* Schizophrenia Research, 2015. **168**(1): p. 161–167.
32. DelBello, M.P., *et al.*, *Prior stimulant treatment in adolescents with bipolar disorder: association with age at onset.* Bipolar Disorders, 2001. **3**(2): p. 53–57.

33. Hollis, C., *et al.*, *Methylphenidate and the risk of psychosis in adolescents and young adults: a population-based cohort study.* The Lancet Psychiatry, 2019. **6**(8): p. 651–658.
34. Cherland, E. and R. Fitzpatrick, *Psychotic side effects of psychostimulants: a 5-year review.* The Canadian Journal of Psychiatry, 1999. **44**(8): p. 811–813.
35. Cressman, A.M., *et al.*, *Prescription stimulant use and hospitalization for psychosis or mania: a population-based study.* Journal of Clinical Psychopharmacology, 2015. **35**(6): p. 667.
36. Castner, S.A. and P.S. Goldman-Rakic, *Long-lasting psychotomimetic consequences of repeated low-dose amphetamine exposure in rhesus monkeys.* Neuropsychopharmacology, 1999. **20**(1): p. 10–28.
37. Castner, S.A. and P.S. Goldman-Rakic, *Amphetamine sensitization of hallucinatory-like behaviors is dependent on prefrontal cortex in nonhuman primates.* Biological psychiatry, 2003. **54**(2): p. 105–110.
38. Ney, P.G., *Psychosis in a child, associated with amphetamine administration.* Canadian Medical Association Journal, 1967. **97**(17): p. 1026.
39. Ross, R.G., *Psychotic and manic-like symptoms during stimulant treatment of attention deficit hyperactivity disorder.* American Journal of Psychiatry, 2006. **163**(7): p. 1149–1152.
40. Rashid, J. and S. Mitelman, *Methylphenidate and somatic hallucinations.* Journal of the American Academy of Child and Adolescent Psychiatry, 2007. **46**(8): p. 945–946.
41. Curtin, K., *et al.*, *Increased risk of diseases of the basal ganglia and cerebellum in patients with a history of attention-deficit/hyperactivity disorder.* Neuropsychopharmacology, 2018. **43**(13): p. 2548–2555.
42. del Campo, N., *et al.*, *The roles of dopamine and noradrenaline in the pathophysiology and treatment of attention-deficit/hyperactivity disorder.* Biological Psychiatry, 2011. **69**(12): p. e145-e157.
43. Pies, R.W., *Debunking the two chemical imbalance myths, again.* Psychiatric Times, 2019. **36**(8).
44. Rosa-Neto, P., *et al.*, *Methylphenidate-evoked changes in striatal dopamine correlate with inattention and impulsivity in adolescents with attention deficit hyperactivity disorder.* NeuroImage, 2005. **25**(3): p. 868–876.

45. Advokat, C., *Literature Review: Update on Amphetamine Neurotoxicity and Its Relevance to the Treatment of ADHD.* Journal of Attention Disorders, 2007. **11**(1): p. 8–16.
46. Diaz Heijtz, R., B. Kolb, and H. Forssberg, *Can a therapeutic dose of amphetamine during pre-adolescence modify the pattern of synaptic organization in the brain?* European Journal of Neuroscience, 2003. **18**(12): p. 3394–3399.
47. Castner, S.A. and G.V. Williams, *From vice to virtue: Insights from sensitization in the nonhuman primate.* Progress in Neuro-Psychopharmacology and Biological Psychiatry, 2007. **31**(8): p. 1572–1592.
48. Robinson, T.E. and B. Kolb, *Persistent Structural Modifications in Nucleus Accumbens and Prefrontal Cortex Neurons Produced by Previous Experience with Amphetamine.* The Journal of Neuroscience, 1997. **17**(21): p. 8491.
49. Andreazza, A.C., *et al.*, *DNA damage in rats after treatment with methylphenidate.* Progress in Neuropsychopharmacology and Biological Psychiatry, 2007. **31**(6): p. 1282–1288.
50. Motaghinejad, M., *et al.*, *Effects of acute doses of methylphenidate on inflammation and oxidative stress in isolated hippocampus and cerebral cortex of adult rats.* Journal of Neural Transmission, 2017. **124**(1): p. 121–131.
51. Motaghinejad, M., M. Motevalian, and B. Shabab, *Effects of chronic treatment with methylphenidate on oxidative stress and inflammation in hippocampus of adult rats.* Neuroscience Letters, 2016. **619**: p. 106–113.
52. Moll, G.H., *et al.*, *Early methylphenidate administration to young rats causes a persistent reduction in the density of striatal dopamine transporters.* Journal of Child and Adolescent Psychopharmacology, 2001. **11**(1): p. 15–24.
53. Sadasivan, S., *et al.*, *Methylphenidate exposure induces dopamine neuron loss and activation of microglia in the basal ganglia of mice.* PloS one, 2012. **7**(3).
54. Carlezon, W.A., Jr. and M.J. Thomas, *Biological substrates of reward and aversion: a nucleus accumbens activity hypothesis.* Neuropharmacology, 2009. **56 Suppl 1**(Suppl 1): p. 122–132.
55. Sax, L., *Boys adrift: The five factors driving the growing epidemic of unmotivated boys and underachieving young men.* 2016: Basic Books.

56. Li, Y. and J.A. Kauer, *Repeated exposure to amphetamine disrupts dopaminergic modulation of excitatory synaptic plasticity and neurotransmission in nucleus accumbens.* Synapse, 2004. **51**(1): p. 1–10.
57. Marco, E.M., *et al.*, *Neurobehavioral adaptations to methylphenidate: the issue of early adolescent exposure.* Neuroscience & Biobehavioral Reviews, 2011. **35**(8): p. 1722–1739.
58. Bolanos, C.A., *et al.*, *Methylphenidate treatment during pre-and periadolescence alters behavioral responses to emotional stimuli at adulthood.* Biological Psychiatry, 2003. **54**(12): p. 1317–1329.
59. Carlezon Jr, W.A., S.D. Mague, and S.L. Andersen, *Enduring behavioral effects of early exposure to methylphenidate in rats.* Biological Psychiatry, 2003. **54**(12): p. 1330–1337.
60. Steiner, H. and V. Van Waes, *Addiction-related gene regulation: risks of exposure to cognitive enhancers vs. other psychostimulants.* Progress in Neurobiology, 2013. **100**: p. 60–80.
61. Lambert, N.M. *Stimulant treatment as a risk factor for nicotine use and substance abuse.* 1998.
62. Quansah, E., *Molecular and Neurochemical Effects of Methylphenidate on the Developing Brain, Thesis submitted in partial fulfilment of the requirements for the degree of Doctor of Philosophy.* 2017, De Montfort University, United Kingdom.
63. Quansah, E. and T.S.C. Zetterström, *Chronic methylphenidate preferentially alters catecholamine protein targets in the parietal cortex and ventral striatum.* Neurochemistry International, 2019. **124**: p. 193–199.
64. Wang, G.-J., *et al.*, *Long-term stimulant treatment affects brain dopamine transporter level in patients with attention deficit hyperactive disorder.* PloS one, 2013. **8**(5).
65. Proebstl, L., *et al.*, *Effects of stimulant drug use on the dopaminergic system: A systematic review and meta-analysis of in vivo neuroimaging studies.* European Psychiatry, 2019. **59**: p. 15–24.
66. Kantak, K.M. and L.P. Dwoskin, *Necessity for research directed at stimulant type and treatment-onset age to access the impact of medication on drug abuse vulnerability in teenagers with ADHD.* Pharmacology Biochemistry and Behavior, 2016. **145**: p. 24.

67. Madjar, N., *et al.*, *Childhood methylphenidate adherence as a predictor of antidepressants use during adolescence.* European Child & Adolescent Psychiatry, 2019: p. 1–9.
68. Vastag, B., *Pay Attention: Ritalin Acts Much Like Cocaine.* JAMA, 2001. **286**(8): p. 905–906.
69. Farrell, M., *et al.*, *Responding to global stimulant use: challenges and opportunities.* The Lancet, 2019. **394**(10209): p. 1652–1667.

❝

"The authors declared no potential conflicts of interest with respect to the research, authorship, and/or publication of this article."

Merzon, Manor, et al. (2020). *ADHD as a Risk Factor for Infection with Covid-19*. Journal of Attention Disorders, 25(13), 1783–1790 [1]

Chapter 12
Can we trust the biomedical consensus? Biases and conflicts of interests

Upon reaching the final chapter of Part Two, some readers probably wonder how it is possible that the public is unaware of the massive evidence against the efficacy and safety of stimulant medications. Does my family doctor not know about the risk for psychotic reaction (Chapter 11) or the increase in Attention Deficit Hyperactivity Disorder (ADHD) symptoms documented in the Multimodal Treatment of ADHD (MTA) study (Chapter 9)? To begin answering these questions, I recommend visiting the official webpage of the National Institute of Mental Health (NIMH) dedicated to "questions and answers" about the institute's seminal project (i.e., the MTA study) [2]. Although this webpage has been revised in November 2009, it mainly presents findings from 1999, which were favorable towards the medications [3]. For some reason, the content of the webpage does not include the unfavorable results that were obtained in the years that followed [e.g., 4, 5].

Well, perhaps the authors of the NIMH webpage were also not aware (like I was before entering the field) of the unfavorable findings that emerged in the long-term studies described in Chapter 9? A close look through the webpage reveals that this option is improbable. At the bottom of the page, under the last question: "Where can I find more information about the MTA study?," the authors provide a "selection of MTA references", which includes some of the studies presented in Chapter 9, including the study from 2009 that reported unfavorable evidence regarding the medications, based on the 8-year-long follow-up of the MTA participants [5]. It is therefore more reasonable to assume that the authors of the NIMH webpage did know about the unfavorable results but chose not to mention them explicitly in their publicly available communications.

Economic interests

How is it possible that such a respected institute conceals such valuable information? With great caution, I propose a one-word answer to this question: 'money' (a three-word answer would probably be: 'loads of money'). In the US, for example, as mentioned in Chapter 7, the pharmacological treatments for ADHD rank at the top of the best-selling drugs for children, especially for boys. According to a study published in *Pediatrics* (a well-established medical journal), for about every ten young boys aged 6–12, there is one boy who receives prescribed stimulant medications [6]. The prevalence of stimulant prescriptions in this study surpassed all other medications (except respiratory agents) given to young children.

Adolescents, as well, use (and abuse) stimulant medications in high rates. Methylphenidate, for example, won the first-place in the 2010 'medication race', with the greatest prescription rates among adolescents aged 12–17 [7]. These high rates are also reflected in concrete medical expenditures. A retrospective study of over three million children found that stimulant medications accounted for the greatest proportion of spending in pediatric medicine [8]. Some might perceive these high rates as a positive indication for the growing public awareness of the need to treat ADHD medically. Others, like the well-acknowledged medical investigative journalists Robert Whitaker and Alan Schwarz, raise concerns that the high prevalence of stimulant use is a product of massive (and ethically questionable) marketing efforts of pharmaceutical companies, which have very little commitment to objective science and actual medical needs [9-11].

A study that tracked the money spent on the marketing of ADHD medications in the US found that between 2014 and 2018, pharmaceutical companies spent over US$20 million on food, beverages, and other presents to 55,105 pediatricians, psychiatrists, and family physicians [12]. I have no doubt that most physicians prescribing these medications do so out of genuine professional considerations. It is clear to me that when a physician is prescribing a medication, he or she believes that its benefits outweigh its risks. However, there is empirical evidence that presents sell drugs. Free meals that are sponsored by pharmacological companies to promote a particular brand of drug are quickly converted to an actual growth in the number of prescriptions written for that drug [13]. Physicians may believe that they are advancing the interests of their patients, but in reality, many of them are infected (even if it is without their knowledge) by the economic interests of the pharma industry [14].

Scientific misconduct

Disturbingly, even scientists who are committed, by the very nature of the profession, to conduct objective research, are sometimes influenced by the interests of the pharma industry [15]. Many of the experts representing the scientific consensus on ADHD currently have, or have had in the past, economic relationships with pharmaceutical companies [see, for example, the long list of conflicts of interests in the 2019 European Consensus Statement; 16]. Some leaders of the consensus, as mentioned in the Introduction, have even failed to declare these problematic relationships [17, 18]. Indeed, the existence of conflicts of interest does not necessarily mean that the resultant scientific research is corrupted, but it certainly requires us to be careful when we interpret its findings.

The reality is that numerous studies in psychiatry are fully, or partially, funded by the pharma industry, and that multiple researchers worked for, or consulted for, pharmacological companies [10, 11]. These inherent conflicts of interest tamper the neutrality and objectivity necessary for conducting reliable scientific research [19, 20], and inevitably lead to poor quality studies with a high risk of bias [21]. Biases can take various forms and shapes [22] — some can be very blatant, as shown in Part Two — but I wish to start our inquiry with the seemingly benign bias, known as *publication bias*. A recent meta-analysis, for example, which sought to demonstrate the (short-term) benefits of methylphenidate beyond multiple studies, also found significant indications for the existence of a publication bias in the relevant literature [23]. Publication bias is a well-acknowledged problematic phenomenon, in which pro-medications articles that report desirable outcomes are submitted and accepted to academic journals, whereas challenging findings, which do not align with the authors'/editors' a priori position, are dismissed and rejected [24].

Indeed, publication bias is a known hurdle plaguing many fields of research. However, in the field of ADHD, this problem relates not only to the loyalty of the authors/editors to a specific school of thought, but also to the inherent conflicts of interest mentioned above. In too many cases, funders inflict explicit pressure on researchers to suppress or delay submissions of studies that do not match their financial goals [25]; but even when the pressure is not explicit, how can we expect researchers, who receive funding from a given company, to report unfavorable results regarding the company's product [26]? This simple truth seems to cause noble scientists (even if unintentionally) to perform a range of manipulations and misrepresentations in their psychiatric research in general [27, 28] and their research on ADHD in particular [22]. The biases are ubiquitous. The vast majority of the 260 studies reviewed by the Cochrane organization (Chapter 10) were rated by independent judges as very poor quality studies (GRADE quality score = very low), with a critical risk of bias [21] — the highest bias score in the measure used to assess its existence [29]. Such a risk comes at a price. When comparing studies funded by pharmaceutical companies with non-funded studies, we learn that the former report significantly fewer adverse outcomes and risks resulting from medication use [21].

The firm grip the pharma industry has on the medical research is terrifying. There are plentiful testimonies that pharma companies operate in similar ways to that of organized crime, including the use of bribery and intimidations as well as the acceptance of the necessary 'side-effects' of killing and deaths [14]. However, even if readers prefer to dismiss these testimonies as unfounded accusations (I can understand that as the truth in this case is too scary to grasp), I urge them not to dismiss the numerous distortions and misrepresentations that have been reviewed in this book. Here is a partial list of places where I presented evidence of such (intentional or unintentional) biases and manipulations:

- The tendentious (and aggressive) wording of the International Consensus Statement presented in the Introduction
- The subtle, yet dramatic, softening of the dysfunction criterion in the *Diagnostic and Statistical Manual of Mental Disorders* (*DSM*) discussed in Chapter 3

- The detached highlights in the adverse outcomes review [30] shown in Chapter 4
- The unfounded messages to clinicians by brain researchers [31], the dismissal of artifact effects of medications on the brain [32], and the publication biases in the literature on brain differences and the literature on genetic differences [33, 34] presented in Chapter 6
- The narrative spin in the meta-analysis on the effects of the medications on functional outcomes [35] analyzed in Chapter 9
- The underestimation and concealment of adverse outcomes of medications in the double-blind controlled study on preschool children [36] and the official consumer leaflet of Ritalin exposed in Chapter 10
- The exclusion of half of the dataset in the Swedish study that addressed the medication-related risk for psychosis [37] uncovered in Chapter 11
- The omission of medication-related information in the 2021 study on COVID-related outcomes [38] discussed in Chapter 11, and the distortions in the 2020 study on the 'protective' role of the medications against COVID-19 infections [1], presented in Chapter 9 (and which will next be discussed in length).

The case study of ADHD and COVID-19

The last example of the 2020 study on COVID-19 infections is in fact a fascinating illustration of the various questionable practices that can be utilized (intentionally or unintentionally) to form the false impressions discussed in Chapters 4 and 9, that is: (1) the impression that ADHD *increases* the risk for future dangers and (2) the impression that daily use of stimulant medications *decreases* the risk for these dangers. Despite the authors' declaration stated in the opening quote of this chapter, according to which they have "no potential conflicts of interest", their study strings together a multi-layered series of scientific distortions and biases.

On July 22, 2020, not long after the first wave of the COVID-19 pandemic, researchers from Israel published a highly concerning article, in which they warned that "ADHD may be a risk factor for COVID-19 infection, independently of other risk factors" [1, p. 1788]. Individuals with ADHD, the researchers hypothesized, are more active and less compliant than others. They probably struggle more than their peers with COVID-19 regulations (e.g., wearing masks, staying at home during lockdowns) and are therefore at a greater risk to be infected by the virus. Complementing this warning, the authors advise individuals with ADHD to adhere to their prescribed medications, since medication use was found in the study to have a protective role "in the attenuation of COVID-19 transmission" (page 1788).

Not surprisingly, these conclusions quickly turned to news headlines. The study, which was based on solid medical records of 14,022 individuals registered in 'Leumit' (a large health service in Israel), and received the 'Kosher stamp' of the *Journal of Attention Disorders,* the home for ADHD research (founded by none other than Keith Conners), attracted considerable public attention (as of October 2021, more than a year after its first publication, the study was still listed as one of the three most read articles in the journal). But how valid are the conclusions of this study? Are individuals with ADHD, unknowingly, contributing to the spread of the pandemic? Should parents of children diagnosed with ADHD hurry to give them stimulant medications even during periods when schools are closed, to protect them from the virus, or to attenuate its spread?

I admit that when I first encountered the headlines regarding this study, I automatically thought that something smelled fishy. Yet, I did not want to dismiss the study based on my own intuitive bias, especially considering the authors' declaration, according to which they have no conflicts of interest. I therefore asked my highly talented friend and colleague, Dr. Yaffa Shir-Raz, to conduct a thorough review of this study with me. We first requested the authors of the study (through a third, neutral person who is not identified as a critic of ADHD), on two separate occasions during August 2020, to give us access to the raw dataset of the study so we could run the required statistical analyses ourselves. Regrettably, we were not granted this access, despite the authors' explicit declaration that "all the data related to this study can be accessed following approval of Leumit health services". [1, p. 1788]. We are still trying to receive access to the data directly from the scientific authority of Leumit health service, but at the time of this writing (April 2022), almost two years after our first contact with the authors, this access has not been granted to us.

Our analysis of the study was therefore based on a careful inspection of the authors' methodological and representational choices, as well as on a comparison of these choices with the methods and results of two additional studies, which were published by the same first author (and additional same co-authors) in the same week. One of these studies, which addressed the relationship between ADHD and a bacterial disease called shigellosis was published in the *very same* journal [39] and one of these studies, which addressed the relationship between vitamin D and COVID-19 symptoms, relied on the *very same* dataset of 14,022 medical records [40].

Our findings from this investigative process can be divided into two main types of biases: (1) manipulations of operational definitions of examined variables; and (2) misrepresentations of data and results. Below I discuss just three sample biases, to provide readers with a glimpse into the various 'scientific' methods used to achieve desirable conclusions, but I encourage the reader to read our entire article that describes the wide range of manipulations and spins occurring in the study [22].

<u>Manipulations of variables</u>

The *first manipulation* occurred in a primary variable of the study, that is the very definition for ADHD. At a first glance, the operational definition of ADHD seems highly reasonable. A person with ADHD is defined as such if he or she had ever been medically diagnosed with the disorder. Imagine how surprised we were when we found out that, in the shigellosis study, which, if you recall, was written by the same first author (and two additional same co-authors), a person with ADHD was categorized as such only if, besides the diagnosis, he or she obtained at least three documented prescriptions for ADHD medications. Why did the researchers choose a different definition for each study? After all, both studies were based on a trustworthy source of data from 'Leumit' (in which medical records of ADHD should be reliable); and both were published more or less at the same time in the very same scientific journal. In the final production, the two studies even appeared together, in the same volume of the journal, one after the other (pp. 1783–1790 and pp. 1791–1800).

In order to answer this question, it is worth reading closely what the authors write in the shigellosis study: The diagnosis of ADHD, they explain, is "given temporally with referral of the patient to ADHD clinic" [39, p. 1792]. In other words, the preliminary diagnosis by itself, according to the researchers themselves, is an unreliable operational definition for ADHD. Why, then, do the very same authors use this problematic definition in their study on ADHD and COVID-19 infections? It is important to understand that we are not engaging in a petty focus on details. Once the researchers chose different definitions for ADHD, huge and unexplained gaps were created between the rates of the diagnoses. While the shigellosis study reported that ADHD rates ranged from 8.6% to 10.6% among children aged 5-18, the COVID-19 study reported that ADHD rates ranged from 18.85% to 28.14% among those aged 5–20 (weighted average for this age group = 20.25%!).

Such prevalence rates are anomalous at an Olympic level. Not only are these estimates double those reported by the same researchers, but they also do not align with the conventional, known rates of the disorder (see Chapter 2), as described by Merzon and colleagues themselves in the introduction to their 2021 study on COVID-19 outcomes. In their words, ADHD is known to have "an estimated worldwide pooled prevalence of between 5% and 7.5% in school aged children and 4.4% in adults" [38, p. 492]. In practice, when such an anomalous number is obtained, it should serve as a warning sign that something is off in the study. Alternatively, if this number is accurate, then it should become the prominent result of the study and be turned into an urgent subject of discussion in the scientific community. Either way, if the basic variable of the research is unreliable, then the entire study is invalid (Box 1, Chapter

1), and if the basic variable is accurate, then it means that we are facing an unexplainable neuropsychiatric epidemic (of ADHD), which may be even more concerning than the coronavirus epidemic.

A *second manipulation* was identified in another primary variable of the study, that is the medication treatment. The authors defined medication treatment by documenting those "who purchased at least three consecutive prescriptions of ADHD medications during the past 12 months" (page 1784). This raises two problems: First, this operational definition (or a similar one), could have been used to define the very existence of ADHD (as chosen in the shigellosis study) — a definition that would have altered the results altogether, since this operational variable was found to 'protect' against COVID-19 infections. Second, this "12 months" operational definition is not suitable to the current study because its outcome measure (positive testing for COVID-19) was confined to a 3-months period only. As mentioned in Chapter 9, no one argues that medications may cure ADHD. The 'therapeutic' and calming effects of the medications only last between 4-12 hours [41] and once the effects fade, the symptoms usually return (some users may even experience a 'rebound effect'). Even the most devoted proponents of the medications would not claim that past usage of stimulant medications (e.g., 9-11 months ago) can be relied on for current management of ADHD symptoms. On the contrary, the European scientific consensus (which includes the corresponding author of the study at hand) is that ADHD is a lifelong condition, which requires regular medical management [16].

Therefore, there is no reason to assume that medications, taken several months before the outbreak of the pandemic, could have reduced the person's current behaviors that led to his/her COVID-19 infection. A much more reasonable methodological decision would be to define 'treated individuals' according to their current usage of medications (e.g., purchasing prescription medications during the confined 3-month period of the study, or perhaps one month before that). The fact that the eventually chosen operational definition included an arbitrary period of time (12 months) that does not align with the general framework of the study, raises an uncomfortable feeling that the dataset was deployed (even if unintentionally) to produce specific results. And even these, unreliable results did not receive adequate presentation, as shown next.

Misrepresentations of data and results

Surely, when the entire research protocol is based on unreliable variables, as illustrated before, its actual results have very little scientific value (Box 1, Chapter 1). However, authors may still present these results in an objective and transparent way that will allow the reader to evaluate their clinical significance. Unfortunately, that was not the case in the study at hand. In addition to the inappropriate definitions of the variables of the study, we identified at least four narrative spins in the presentation of the results, both in the abstract, and in the body, of the study. The concept of "spin" might perhaps strike you as pertinent only in the political/public sphere, but in recent years, with the increase of distortions in medical science, it has begun to be used in leading scientific journals, to describe unwanted practices that are intended to achieve desired outcomes by questionable means [42]. Below is a particularly disturbing example of such a spin.

Towards the end of the article, the researchers note "a major weakness" of the study and admit that "data regarding the presenting symptoms and severity of COVID-19 infection, as well as adverse clinical outcomes (hospitalization and mechanical ventilation) were not assessed" (page 1788). This choice of words ("not assessed") is, in fact, quite problematic. After all, the authors had access to medical records, which included, according to their own words, "medical visits, laboratory tests, hospitalizations, and medication prescriptions" (page 1784). Furthermore, in the study that dealt with vitamin D and COVID-19, which was based precisely on the same dataset of 14,022 medical records, and which had three of the same authors, the researchers did assess the symptoms and severity of COVID-19 infection [40]. Finally, in their 2021 study [38], which addressed the same topic (ADHD and COVID-19) and relied on an overlapping dataset, the authors specifically targeted these severe outcomes of the COVID-19 infections (while failing to report of different outcomes — the outcomes of the medications for ADHD, as discussed in Chapter 11).

Why did the researchers choose not to assess these complications in the 2020 study if they had the data and why did they choose not to mention the role of the medications in their 2021 study? These are crucial questions because, without this information, we cannot evaluate the safety of the medications for ADHD. Is it proper to prescribe ADHD medications during an active pandemic? We know from Chapter 11 that stimulant use might trigger cardiovascular complications [e.g., 43], and that cardiovascular complications are a strong risk factor for severe outcomes of COVID-19 [44, 45]. Correspondingly, we remember the newly released European Guidelines, which determined that ADHD medications should not be started during the pandemic if the person has a history of breathing and/or cardiovascular-related problems [46]. Finally, we learn from studies on neurotoxins, such as methamphetamines, that psychostimulants can alter the blood-brain barrier permeability, thus perhaps increasing the risk for invasion of dangerous viruses into the brain [47, 48]. There is also some evidence that prohibited stimulant drugs [49], as well as medically prescribed stimulant medications for ADHD [50, 51] may have a negative impact on our natural immune system. In light of these warnings, as well as the known adverse outcomes of stimulant medications (Chapters 10 and 11), the authors should have ruled out the possibility that the medications are actually **not** safe for individuals infected with the coronavirus. Their questionable methodological and representational choices have, literally, life and death implications.

Amazingly, not only did the authors not report/analyze the severe outcomes of COVID-19 in their 2020 study, they also cite the above European guidelines as if they served as proof for their own recommendation. Here is the precise wording in which the authors framed their recommendation: "Adherence to anti-ADHD treatment should be encouraged in an attempt to reduce the spread of COVID-19 infection (Cortese *et al.*, 2020)." This is a noteworthy spin, because the guidelines that are quoted in this sentence by Prof. Samuele Cortese and colleagues [46] suggest the exact opposite — that ADHD medications may **not** be appropriate in times of respiratory pandemic, because of their potential adverse outcomes. Perhaps this is why the authors chose **not** to present the effects of the medications in their 2021 study — Prof. Cortese, the first author of the guidelines joined them as a co-author in this study on severe outcomes of COVID-19 [38]. De facto, the authors' choices left us with the suspicious situation described in Chapter 11, whereby the 2020 study reporting of medications did not report of severe COVID outcomes and the 2021 study reporting of severe COVID outcomes did not report of medication use. Readers can only wonder what underlies these misrepresentations. Is it possible that stimulant use increases the risk for COVID-19 symptoms and hospitalizations?

The pharmaceutical industry

Manipulations, misrepresentations, and sometimes actual frauds, aimed to distort information regarding medications, such as the ones described above, are not new to biomedicine [26, 52, 53]. Previous reviews have shown similar biases in multiple biomedical studies, including for example: Ignoring contradicting results [42]; reducing data in a biased fashion; ignoring adverse outcomes, inappropriate subgroup analyses; and selective reporting of subgroup and outcomes [54]. Earlier studies also warned against the potential ramifications of such distortions and their biased impact on clinicians and patients [56, 56], and suggested valuable scientific practices (e.g., register and share datasets with the scientific community) that could reduce these biases [57, 58]. However, the field of attention disorders, as mentioned above, seems particularly vulnerable to such malpractices because of the enmeshed relationships with the pharmaceutical industry and the large sums of money that are involved [9, 10].

Indeed, the authors of the COVID-19 studies discussed above "declared no potential conflicts of interest" and I assume that this was indeed the case. However, the influence of the pharma companies may still be present, even if not explicitly. First, the corresponding author of these studies had declared, in the near past [see in: 16], that she served on the counseling and advisory boards of leading pharma companies, such as Janssen-Cilag, Teva, and Novartis. Similarly, three authors of the 2020 study who declared "no potential conflicts" [1] provided an "author note" in their 2021 study [38, pp. 498–499], in which they reported of personal fees, or of reimbursements for travel and accommodation expenses, from pharmaceutical companies (I am not sure why this information was not disclosed in the 2020 study and how it is possible that the authors could still declare "no potential conflicts of interest" in their 2021 study, when their "author note" implies otherwise). Second, the accumulation of so many blatant distortions and discrepancies in these studies leaves the impartiality of the authors open to question. Third, during the beginning of the COVID-19 crisis, the sales of ADHD medications had probably declined. As described in Chapter 3, during the first COVID lockdown, many parents (at least, in Israel) discontinued their children's medication treatment [59]. This potential reduction may also be reflected in the authors' own study from 2020, in which only a quarter of the diagnosed individuals (24.6%) purchased at least three consecutive ADHD-medication-prescriptions [1].

For those who are not deeply involved in empirical-quantitative research, this claim regarding the pervasive influence of the pharma industry may sound like a conspiracy theory. However, the unpleasant truth is that biomedical research has been infected with severe distortions [42, 52], which can mainly be explained through the impact of the industry [14, 28]. This is one of the reasons why sharing raw datasets, whenever it is ethically possible, is highly encouraged [58]. Nevertheless, as illustrated above, not all researchers comply with this basic transparency requirement. In our efforts to receive access to the dataset used in the aforementioned COVID-19 studies, we encountered a range of stalling tactics, which seemed to have led the editor-in-chief of the *Journal of Attention Disorders* to propose that we submit a new article that will summarize our concerns with these studies. We have actually accepted his invitation, but after the peer-review process he informed us that the journal is "not the best placement" for our article, despite its specific focus on studies that were published in this journal and despite his final judgment that our article is: "worthy of publication". We therefore submitted this article to a different (great) academic journal and readers are highly encouraged to read it as it provides a rare glimpse into the scientific 'sausage factory', where biases and misconducts substitute for research integrity and transparency [60].

And if academic scholars are falling prey to dishonesty, what can we expect from researchers who work directly for the pharmaceutical companies? There is accumulating evidence (e.g., from the US legal system), that companies, which market psychiatric medications, manipulate their data to achieve desirable results and hide unfavorable results that undermine the efficacy or the safety of their products [11, 14]. Their final publications may seem transparent and purely scientific, but de facto, they comprise designated distortions that misrepresent their data and mislead their customers [28]. "Drug companies", according to Professor Emeritus of psychiatry, Allen Frances — the honorable head of the task force developing the fourth edition of the *DSM* — "were given the means, the motive, and the message to disease-monger ADHD and blow it up out of all proportion" [61]. In other words, even believers of the disorder, such as Frances who supervised the creation of the *DSM*, are worried that the pharma industry is corrupting the scientific grounding of ADHD. The "drug companies", in his words, "succeeded beyond all expectations in achieving a triumph of clever advertising over common sense".

At this point, it is important to me to repeat my earlier statement that, in the context of the problematic relationships between the pharmaceutical companies and the physicians/scientists, I **do not** suggest that the latter are acting with malicious intent. I am positive that most scientists and practitioners believe that the medications they are researching, or prescribing, are required for the improvement of the quality of life of individuals diagnosed with ADHD. But even they, perhaps more than others, are subjected to the influence of the powerful marketing campaigns of the large pharmaceutical companies [9]. Thus, ultimately, the scientific medical information that reaches the public, who is not familiar with these problematic power dynamics, and not trained in complex academic readings, is severely corrupted.

In my view, the conflicts of interest that exist between pharmaceutical companies and scientists, as well as the host of risks involved in providing pharmacological treatments (Chapters 10 and 11), place a great deal of responsibility on physicians. The consumer leaflet, as shown in the previous chapters, is an insufficient and inaccurate source of information, to say the least (Figure 3, Chapter 10). Some might even say that, like the above examples for misrepresentations, the leaflet is specifically structured to downplay the adverse outcomes of the medications (Chapter 10). It is therefore crucial that physicians, who prescribe medications for ADHD, would provide patients with a decent amount of information regarding the known risks of the medications. The list of adverse outcomes is quite long and serious, as discussed in Chapters 10 and 11, and physicians who are reluctant to share parts of this list with their patients should at least consider informing their patients about the existence of the historical debate over the validity of ADHD (Part One), and over the legitimacy of treating it with stimulant medications (Part Two).

Medical ethics and plain human morality require that.

Primum non nocere.

First, do no harm.

References

1. Merzon, E., *et al., ADHD as a Risk Factor for Infection With Covid-19.* Journal of Attention Disorders, 2020. **25**(13): p. 1783–1790.
2. NIMH, *The Multimodal Treatment of Attention Deficit Hyperactivity Disorder Study (MTA):Questions and Answers.* 2009, National Institute of Mental Health (NIMH) website. Last retrieved on September 23, 2021 from: https://www.nimh.nih.gov/funding/clinical-research/practical/mta/the-multimodal-treatment-of-attention-deficit-hyperactivity-disorder-study-mtaquestions-and-answers#Molina.

3. The MTA Cooperative Group, *A 14-month randomized clinical trial of treatment strategies for attention-deficit/hyperactivity disorder.* Archives of general psychiatry, 1999. **56**(12): p. 1073–1086.
4. Jensen, P.S., *et al., 3-year follow-up of the NIMH MTA study.* Journal of the American Academy of Child & Adolescent Psychiatry, 2007. **46**(8): p. 989–1002.
5. Molina, B.S.G., *et al., The MTA at 8 years: prospective follow-up of children treated for combined-type ADHD in a multisite study.* Journal of the American Academy of Child & Adolescent Psychiatry, 2009. **48**(5): p. 484–500.
6. Qato, D.M., *et al., Prescription Medication Use Among Children and Adolescents in the United States.* Pediatrics, 2018. **142**(3): p. e20181042.
7. Chai, G., *et al., Trends of Outpatient Prescription Drug Utilization in US Children, 2002–2010.* Pediatrics, 2012. **130**(1): p. 23.
8. Cohen, E., *et al., High-Expenditure Pharmaceutical Use Among Children in Medicaid.* Pediatrics, 2017. **140**(3): p. e20171095.
9. Schwarz, A., *ADHD nation: Children, doctors, big pharma, and the making of an American epidemic.* 2017: Simon and Schuster.
10. Whitaker, R. and L. Cosgrove, *Psychiatry under the influence: Institutional corruption, social injury, and prescriptions for reform.* 2015: Springer.
11. Whitaker, R., *Anatomy of an epidemic: Psychiatric drugs and the astonishing rise of mental illness in America.* Ethical Human Psychology and Psychiatry, 2005. **7**(1): p. 23.
12. Hadland, S.E., *et al., Analysis of Pharmaceutical Industry Marketing of Stimulants, 2014 Through 2018.* JAMA Pediatrics, 2020. **174**(4): p. 385–387.
13. DeJong, C., *et al., Pharmaceutical Industry–Sponsored Meals and Physician Prescribing Patterns for Medicare Beneficiaries.* JAMA Internal Medicine, 2016. **176**(8): p. 1114–1122.
14. Gotzsche, P., *Deadly Medicines and Organised Crime: How Big Pharma Has Corrupted Healthcare.* Radcliffe, London and New York, 2013.
15. Lenzer, J., *Why we can't trust clinical guidelines.* BMJ, 2013. **346**: p. f3830.
16. Kooij, J.J.S., *et al., Updated European Consensus Statement on diagnosis and treatment of adult ADHD.* European Psychiatry, 2019. **56**: p. 14–34.
17. Lenzer, J., *Review launched after Harvard psychiatrist failed to disclose industry funding.* BMJ, 2008. **336**(7657): p. 1327.

18. Harris, G. and B. Carey, *Researchers fail to reveal full drug pay*, in *New York Times*. 2008, New York Times, Last retrieved on August 26, 2021 from: https://www.nytimes.com/2008/06/08/us/08conflict.html.
19. Jureidini, J. and L.B. McHenry, *The illusion of evidence based medicine*. BMJ, 2022. **376**: p. o702.
20. Howick, J., *Exploring the asymmetrical relationship between the power of finance bias and evidence*. Perspectives in biology and medicine, 2019. **62**(1): p. 159–187.
21. Storebø, O.J., *et al.*, *Methylphenidate for attention deficit hyperactivity disorder (ADHD) in children and adolescents–assessment of adverse events in non-randomised studies*. Cochrane Database of Systematic Reviews, 2018(5).
22. Ophir, Y. and Y. Shir-Raz, *Manipulations and Spins in Attention Disorders Research: The Case of ADHD and COVID-19*. Ethical Human Psychology and Psychiatry, 2020. **22**: p. 98–113.
23. Pievsky, M.A. and R.E. McGrath, *Neurocognitive effects of methylphenidate in adults with attention-deficit/hyperactivity disorder: A meta-analysis*. Neuroscience & Biobehavioral Reviews, 2018. **90**: p. 447–455.
24. Dickersin, K., *et al.*, *Publication bias and clinical trials*. Controlled Clinical Trials, 1987. **8**(4): p. 343–353.
25. McCrabb, S., *et al.*, *"He who pays the piper calls the tune": Researcher experiences of funder suppression of health behaviour intervention trial findings*. PloS one, 2021. **16**(8): p. e0255704.
26. Ritchie, S., *Science fictions: How fraud, bias, negligence, and hype undermine the search for truth*. 2020: Metropolitan Books.
27. Cosgrove, L., *et al.*, *Financial ties between DSM-IV panel members and the pharmaceutical industry*. Psychotherapy and Psychosomatics, 2006. **75**(3): p. 154–160.
28. Whitaker, R., *Anatomy of an Industry: Commerce, Payments to Psychiatrists and Betrayal of the Public Good*. 2021, Mad in America. Last retrieved on September 28, 2021, from: https://www.madinamerica.com/2021/09/anatomy-industry-commerce-payments-psychiatrists-betrayal-public-good/?fbclid=IwAR2xyMWzXnl9gj5zcb8i-W-Sv0Uw2nznx5WcZfql4COozFweJrNeiPEErr8.

29. Sterne, J.A.C., *et al., ROBINS-I: a tool for assessing risk of bias in non-randomised studies of interventions.* BMJ, 2016. **355**: p. i4919.
30. Nigg, J.T., *Attention-deficit/hyperactivity disorder and adverse health outcomes.* Clinical Psychology Review, 2013. **33**(2): p. 215–228.
31. Hoogman, M., *et al., Subcortical brain volume differences in participants with attention deficit hyperactivity disorder in children and adults: a cross-sectional mega-analysis.* The Lancet Psychiatry, 2017. **4**(4): p. 310–319.
32. Spencer, T.J., *et al., In vivo neuroreceptor imaging in attention-deficit/hyperactivity disorder: a focus on the dopamine transporter.* Biological Psychiatry, 2005. **57**(11): p. 1293–1300.
33. Bobb, A.J., *et al., Molecular genetic studies of ADHD: 1991 to 2004.* American Journal of Medical Genetics Part B: Neuropsychiatric Genetics, 2006. **141B**(6): p. 551–565.
34. Samea, F., *et al., Brain alterations in children/adolescents with ADHD revisited: A neuroimaging meta-analysis of 96 structural and functional studies.* Neuroscience & Biobehavioral Reviews, 2019.
35. Boland, H., *et al., A literature review and meta-analysis on the effects of ADHD medications on functional outcomes.* Journal of Psychiatric Research, 2020. **123**: p. 21–30.
36. Firestone, P., *et al., Short-term side effects of stimulant medication are increased in preschool children with attention-deficit/hyperactivity disorder: a double-blind placebo-controlled study.* Journal of Child and Adolescent Psychopharmacology, 1998. **8**(1): p. 13–25.
37. Hollis, C., *et al., Methylphenidate and the risk of psychosis in adolescents and young adults: a population-based cohort study.* The Lancet Psychiatry, 2019. **6**(8): p. 651–658.
38. Merzon, E., *et al., The Association between ADHD and the Severity of COVID-19 Infection.* Journal of Attention Disorders, 2021. **26**(4): p. 491–501.
39. Merzon, E., *et al., Early Childhood Shigellosis and Attention Deficit Hyperactivity Disorder: A Population-Based Cohort Study with a Prolonged Follow-up.* Journal of Attention Disorders, 2020. **25**(13): p. 1791–1800.

40. Merzon, E., *et al.*, *Low plasma 25 (OH) vitamin D level is associated with increased risk of COVID-19 infection: an Israeli population-based study.* The FEBS journal, 2020. **287**(17): p. 3693–3702.
41. Wolraich, M.L. and M.A. Doffing, *Pharmacokinetic Considerations in the Treatment of Attention-Deficit Hyperactivity Disorder with Methylphenidate.* CNS Drugs, 2004. **18**(4): p. 243–250.
42. Boutron, I. and P. Ravaud, *Misrepresentation and distortion of research in biomedical literature.* Proceedings of the National Academy of Sciences, 2018. **115**(11): p. 2613–2619.
43. Amour, M.D.S., *et al.*, *What is the effect of ADHD stimulant medication on heart rate and blood pressure in a community sample of children?* Canadian Journal of Public Health, 2018. **109**(3): p. 395–400.
44. Williamson, E.J., *et al.*, *Factors associated with COVID-19-related death using OpenSAFELY.* Nature, 2020. **584**(7821): p. 430–436.
45. Clerkin, K.J., *et al.*, *COVID-19 and cardiovascular disease.* Circulation, 2020. **141**(20): p. 1648–1655.
46. Cortese, S., *et al.*, *Starting ADHD medications during the COVID-19 pandemic: recommendations from the European ADHD Guidelines Group.* The Lancet Child & Adolescent Health, 2020. **4**(6): p. e15.
47. Kousik, S.M., T.C. Napier, and P.M. Carvey, *The effects of psychostimulant drugs on blood brain barrier function and neuroinflammation.* Frontiers in Pharmacology, 2012. **3**: p. 121–121.
48. Sajja, R.K., S. Rahman, and L. Cucullo, *Drugs of abuse and blood-brain barrier endothelial dysfunction: A focus on the role of oxidative stress.* Journal of Cerebral Blood Flow & Metabolism, 2016. **36**(3): p. 539–554.
49. Carrico, A.W., *et al.*, *Stimulant use is associated with immune activation and depleted tryptophan among HIV-positive persons on anti-retroviral therapy.* Brain, behavior, and immunity, 2008. **22**(8): p. 1257–1262.
50. Kocaman, C., *et al.*, *Ischemic stroke associated with the use of short term oral methylphenidate.* Gülhane Tip Dergisi, 2006. **48**(3): p. 169.
51. Millichap, J., *Effect of Methylphenidate on the Immune System.* Pediatric Neurology Briefs, 1997. **11**(8).

52. Steen, R.G., *Retractions in the scientific literature: is the incidence of research fraud increasing?* Journal of Medical Ethics, 2011. **37**(4): p. 249–253.
53. Simmons, J.P., L.D. Nelson, and U. Simonsohn, *False-positive psychology: Undisclosed flexibility in data collection and analysis allows presenting anything as significant.* Psychological Science, 2011. **22**(11): p. 1359–1366.
54. Al-Marzouki, S., *et al.*, *The effect of scientific misconduct on the results of clinical trials: a Delphi survey.* Contemporary Clinical Trials, 2005. **26**(3): p. 331–337.
55. Boutron, I., *et al.*, *Impact of spin in the abstracts of articles reporting results of randomized controlled trials in the field of cancer: the SPIIN randomized controlled trial.* Journal of Clinical Oncology, 2014. **32**(36): p. 4120–4126.
56. Boutron, I., *et al.*, *Three randomized controlled trials evaluating the impact of "spin" in health news stories reporting studies of pharmacologic treatments on patients'/caregivers' interpretation of treatment benefit.* BMC Medicine, 2019. **17**(1): p. 105.
57. Stroebe, W., T. Postmes, and R. Spears, *Scientific misconduct and the myth of self-correction in science.* Perspectives on Psychological Science, 2012. **7**(6): p. 670–688.
58. Cumming, G., *The New Statistics: Why and How.* Psychological Science, 2013. **25**(1): p. 7–29.
59. Ophir, Y., *Evidence that the Diagnosis of ADHD Does Not Reflect a Chronic Bio-Medical Disease.* Ethical Human Psychology and Psychiatry, 2022. **23–2**.
60. Ophir, Y. and Y. Shir-Raz, *Discrepancies in Studies on ADHD and COVID-19 Raise Concerns Regarding the Risks of Stimulant Treatments During an Active Pandemic.* Accepted Manuscript. Ethical Human Psychology and Psychiatry.
61. Leo, J. and J.R. Lacasse, *The New York Times and the ADHD Epidemic.* Society, 2015. **52**(1): p. 3–8.

Interim Summary of Part Two
Nothing like eyeglasses

The medical-scientific picture that emerges from Part Two is bleak. When we quieten the commercial cacophony of the pharma industry, we are left with ineffective, highly dangerous, and potentially addictive drugs. The short-term clinical value of stimulant medications, the first-line treatment for Attention Deficit Hyperactivity Disorder (ADHD), is minor and questionable, and even if the medications do bring some improvement (especially for schoolteachers), the available evidence suggests that they have zero long-term efficacy against symptoms and dangers associated with ADHD. On the contrary, when used for prolonged periods, the medications seem to produce *reverse efficacy*, that is, aggravation of ADHD-related symptoms, Oppositional Defiant Disorder symptoms (a disorder that occurs in high comorbidity with ADHD), and general impairments in functioning.

Under the public radar, massive evidence is also accumulating regarding the non-serious and serious adverse outcomes of these medications. In fact, the term 'non-serious outcomes' is misleading, since it includes growth impairments, Obsessive-Compulsive Disorder-like behaviors, involuntary motor/vocal tics, depression, and many more outcomes that harm the user's quality of life. The desirable effects of the medications (i.e., the suppression of unwanted behaviors and the enhancement of attention abilities) is likely to be a misrepresentation of well-documented adverse effects. The medications cause many children to become socially distant, apathetic, and over-focused on useless activities.

Furthermore, about 1% of the treated population (a large number considering the scope of stimulant use today) suffer even worse adverse outcomes, such as suicide ideation, heart dysregulations, and psychotic or manic episodes – psychiatric reactions that are sometimes wrongly interpreted as signs of prodrome psychiatric disorders, which lead to further pharmacological interventions. As such, the popular treatment of choice for the most common neuropsychiatric label in childhood has become a central gateway to additional psychiatric labels, hospitalizations, and other dangerous psychoactive medications that cross the blood-brain barrier and cause sustainable changes in the brain.

Bearing this information in mind, we can now return to address the popular biomedical-oriented argument according to which individuals with ADHD should use stimulant medications regularly, in the same way people with visual impairments wear eyeglasses, or the way people with chronic diabetes manage their blood sugar levels. The integrative picture that arises from the two parts of this book suggests that this argument is flawed in at least three ways:

1. Even without considering the specific criticism about the validity of ADHD (Part One), the very comparison between organic/bodily conditions, which are typically measured through objective tools (e.g., blood tests), to amorphic psychiatric labels that rely exclusively on subjective assessments of behaviors, is inappropriate and misleading. The chemical imbalance hypothesis and the presumed selective/paradoxical effects of the medications are a myth (Chapter 6). Stimulants do not 'fix' biochemical imbalances and they can easily be used also by non-ADHD individuals (who do not have the alleged brain deficit), to enhance cognitive performance.
2. As opposed to chronic diabetes, visual impairments, or even a temporary fractured leg that restrict the individual's everyday functioning, regardless of school demands, the main impairment in ADHD is manifested in school. Blood sugar supplements/medications, eyeglasses, and walking crutches are all needed outside of school premises as well, even during weekends and holidays. ADHD, in contrast, is a 'seasonal disease'. When schools are closed, its medical management is often no longer needed. This simple fact is even acknowledged, to some extent, in the official Ritalin leaflet, which states that: "During the course of treatment for ADHD, the doctor may tell you to stop taking Ritalin for certain periods of time (e.g., every weekend or school vacations) to see if it is still necessary to take it" (Chapter 9).

Incidentally, these 'treatment breaks', according to the leaflet, "also help prevent a slowdown in growth that sometimes occurs when children take this medicine for a long time" — a noteworthy point that brings us to the third, and most important error in the comparison between stimulant medications and other daily, physical/medical aids.

3. The benign examples used by proponents of the medications, such as eyeglasses or walking crutches are not regulated by the Dangerous Drugs Ordinance. Typically, these medical aids do not cause serious physiological and emotional adverse outcomes. If stimulant drugs are so safe as "experts say" (Chapter 10), like "Tylenol and aspirin" (Chapter 11), why do we insist that they be medically prescribed by licensed physicians? Considering the rebuttal of the myth regarding the selective/paradoxical effect of the medications (Chapter 6), this question has philosophical and societal implications. After all, if the medications are safe and helpful to various populations (i.e., not only to people with ADHD), what is the moral justification to prohibit their usage among non-diagnosed individuals (who were 'unlucky' and had only 5 symptoms, which were not sufficient to meet the 6-symptom threshold of the *Diagnostic and Statistical Manual of Mental Disorders (DSM)*. This is an unjustified discrimination. Moreover, why are we condemning students who use these medications to improve their grades? If regular use of Ritalin and alike is so safe, why not place them on the shelves of the pharmacies, next to the non-prescription pain relievers, moisturizers, and chocolate energy bars?

The last rhetoric questions illustrate how far the eyeglasses and the diabetes metaphors are from the clinical reality and the scientific evidence regarding ADHD and stimulant medications. ADHD medications, as presented in the introductory chapter of Part Two, are not fundamentally different from other psychoactive drugs that cross the blood-brain barrier. At first usage, they may trigger intense sensations of potency or euphoria, but when used for prolonged periods, their desired effects subside, and their unwanted negative effects start to emerge. The brain recognizes the psychoactive substances as neurotoxins and activates a compensatory mechanism in an attempt to fight these harmful invaders. It is this activation of the compensatory mechanism, not the ADHD, that causes the biochemical imbalance in the brain (Chapters 6 and 11). The prolonged usage of stimulant medications is expected to increase the levels of the neurotransmitters transporters and corrupt the receptors of the postsynaptic neurons, thereby leading to physiological addiction. Behavioral conditioning and deterministic messages by adult caregivers may also create a sense of psychological dependency on the drug. Then, when users seek to stop taking these substances, they are likely to exhibit withdrawal symptoms and aggravation of exactly the same behaviors that led to the prescription of the medication in the first place.

Unfortunately, many parents are unaware of this expected drug-tolerance process, and mistakenly assume that this increase of symptoms, when their children are not taking their medications, is a strong sign for the necessity of the medications ("the child must take his medication, otherwise he destroys our home"). Parents are not always aware that this *rebound effect* is actually a warning sign that the child might be developing physiological dependence on the drug.

I recognize that the information presented in Part Two is a lot, and not easy, to digest, but I hope that it will increase parents' awareness and help them break the walls of silence. It's about time, more than forty years after the first introduction of ADHD, that we liberate ourselves from the enticing grasp of the pharmaceutical industry. We live in an age characterized by the democratization of knowledge and unprecedented access to scientific information, and there is no reason for us to allow the drug companies to keep hiding the disturbing information about ADHD and its related, ineffective and unsafe medications.

Now that we know how problematic the treatment of choice for ADHD is, we can return to the primary goal of this book, which is to explore the validity of the allegedly consensual biomedical notions regarding ADHD and its related treatment. The final General Discussion chapter organizes the numerous reliability and validity gaps that were identified throughout this book. By drawing the 'bigger' socioeducational problem, and discussing alternative perspectives and potential solutions, I hope that medical officials will consider the option that ADHD no longer be listed as a legitimate neuropsychiatric illness and that stimulant medications would no longer be given to children as a legitimate, first-line cure.

❝

"We, the undersigned consortium of international scientists, are deeply concerned about the periodic inaccurate portrayal of attention deficit hyperactivity disorder (ADHD) in media reports... We fear that inaccurate stories rendering ADHD as myth, fraud, or benign condition may cause thousands of sufferers not to seek treatment for their disorder... The views of a handful of nonexpert doctors that ADHD does not exist are contrasted against mainstream scientific views... All of the major medical associations and government health agencies recognize ADHD as a genuine disorder."

Barkley, R. A. (2002). *International consensus statement on ADHD*. Journal of the American Academy of Child and Adolescent Psychiatry, 41(12), 1389 [1].

General Discussion
A time to tear down and a time to build

I have deep respect for the authors of the 2002 International Consensus Statement who devoted their lifetime to research inattention and hyperactivity behaviors. I do not doubt their good intentions. I even believe that a small percentage of children derived some benefits from being diagnosed with Attention Deficit Hyperactivity Disorder (ADHD), whether through less judgmental and more compassionate feedback from their caregivers, or through their eligibility for concrete psycho-educational support. However, I respectfully disagree with the consensus members' deterministic biomedical approach. The concern that ADHD is a "myth, fraud, or benign condition" does not emerge simply from "media reports" or "inaccurate stories"; it is voiced by multiple scientists and clinicians (Introduction), and it is anchored in firm empirical evidence, which is now organized and consolidated in one scientific source (this book).

The current General Discussion Chapter provides (1) an integrative summary of the major arguments of this book alongside (2) a representative case study that emphasizes the crucial need for a substantive change. At the heart of this chapter, I chose to (3) assemble all the validity gaps mentioned in this book (N = 75) into one 'mega-table' that tears down the biomedical conceptualization about ADHD and requires its transfer from the medical sphere to the psycho-educational sphere. Correspondingly, the last section of this chapter is dedicated to (4) practical and conceptual directions that could help us build a suitable and empowering environment for our children — one that does not involve (flawed) medical diagnoses and (dangerous) medications.

Brief integrative summary

Despite the biomedical conceptualization of ADHD as a chronic "brain disorder" or as "the diabetes of psychiatry" (Introduction), the neurobiological literature did not yield reliable and clear biological markers that can be used for actual clinical diagnosis in the field (Chapter 6). Moreover, even if clear biological markers were to be found, our basic approach to the mind-body problem (i.e., the monism approach) and the very definition of ADHD as a neuropsychiatric disorder require us to explore the validity of the disorder through the same prism of all other *Diagnostic and Statistical Manual of Mental Disorders* (*DSM*)-based disorders, that is: the "Four Ds" criteria of psychiatric diagnosis (Chapter 1).

At the heart of Part One of this book, we have learned that the theoretical concept of ADHD and its actual applications in real-life settings do not meet the required criteria of Deviance, Dysfunction, Danger, and Distress, especially when school-related considerations are taken out of the diagnostic equation (Chapter 2–5). One prominent example (out of dozens provided in this book) is the ever-changing prevalence rates of the disorder, which depend on almost every sociodemographic parameter possible, and that surged in some places, to inconceivable percentages of over 20% (Chapter 2). Another example is the large percentage of comorbidities, which eliminate any traces of discriminant validity (for a short overview of additional facts that do not align with the biomedical consensus, see the Interim Summary of Part One).

The rebuttal of the conceptualization of ADHD presented in Part One does not mean that I am a 'psychopathology denier' — not at all. A small percentage of children experience considerable distress and major functional difficulties that do meet the required criteria for a mental disorder (and I am doing my best to treat such children in our community mental health center). However, this mental disorder is probably not ADHD (at least, not in its current, softened formulation as an all-inclusive trashcan diagnosis), but a much more severe pathology, which includes explicit symptoms of distress and vivid functional impairments that are not related to school demands (Chapter 5).

I also believe that the remaining millions of perfectly healthy children, who are accidently labeled with ADHD, should receive the maximum support and compassion from their caregivers. We should, by no means, travel back in time and return to call these energetic/distracted children with derogatory names, such as lazy or stupid. However, in the same breath, I insist that these healthy children not be led to believe that something is wrong with their brain. Part One of this book has proven that the clinical diagnosis of ADHD does not reflect a chronic brain disorder that must be treated medically, every day, to prevent its alleged negative outcomes. Perhaps ADHD can be reconsidered as a "mode of thought" (Chapter 6) or a multifaceted personality trait (which has both disadvantages and advantages), but it cannot remain a legitimate medical condition.

Considering the poor validity of the disorder, extra attention should be directed at the legitimacy of its related treatment. Part Two of this book discussed the available evidence regarding the efficacy and safety of stimulant medications (e.g., Ritalin, Adderall) — the first-line pharmacological treatment for ADHD. Although multiple studies suggested that stimulant medications can make children more obedient, focused, and calm in the short term, their conclusions are limited due to poor research quality and a critical risk of bias (Chapters 8 and 12). A literature review of the short-term benefits of the medications revealed that these benefits are almost never converted into valuable and clinically significant positive impacts on the child's overall academic performance or quality of life (Chapter 8). Long-term benefits of the medications are even more questionable, considering the lack of sufficient longitudinal research, and the fact that the longitudinal studies that do exist (e.g., the MTA study by the NIMH) did not yield the expected favorable results regarding the medications' efficacy (Chapter 9).

Not only the medications do not seem to be effective, they are also expected to intensify symptoms of inattention and hyperactivity (Chapter 9), perhaps through the brain compensatory mechanism (Chapter 11). Alongside these ADHD-like symptoms, stimulant medications have a tremendous number of adverse outcomes, including for example, apathy, Obsessive-Compulsive Disorder (OCD)-like manifestations, and depression (Chapter 10). Indeed, adult caregivers may confuse these suppressive side-effects with desirable outcomes (e.g., less disruptions in the classroom), but the sad truth is that these outcomes typically reflect well-documented adverse effects, such as over focus on useless tasks, zombie-like behaviors, isolation from friends, and a significant reduction in pleasure or interests — the hallmarks of depression (Chapter 10). Some children would eventually develop serious adverse conditions (Chapter 11) that are hidden from the public (Chapter 12), including long-term brain changes. The brain recognizes the toxic nature of the medications and operates a compensatory mechanism that eventually disturbs its delicate biochemical balance, and, in some cases, triggers extensive and irreversible changes.

The available research suggests that the medications also increase the risks for addictions, heart dysregulations, and severe mania or psychosis. Unfortunately, these last psychiatric reactions are usually not attributed by medical personnel to the effects of the medications, thus turning the first-line pharmacological treatment for ADHD to a central gateway to further psychoactive treatments and psychiatric hospitalizations. The next section, which comprises a representative case study, illustrates this last point, as well as other major ideas conversed in this book. Following this case study, we can return to the major goals of this chapter, that is: the tearing down of the biomedical construct of ADHD and the building of a child-friendly and drug-free environment.

A representative case study

As we approach the ending of the book, let me tell the story of Toby — a remarkable case-study published in the *Journal of Child and Adolescent Psychopharmacology* [2], which illustrates well how the allegedly harmless labeling of ADHD and its 'safe' pharmacological treatment can trigger a serious, and sometimes irreversible, psychiatric deterioration.

Toby, an energetic and kind-hearted 4th grade student, was born to two healthy parents in a stable relationship, with no history of mental disorders in the family. As a baby, Toby ate and slept well and was generally quite easy. However, when he entered kindergarten at the age of 3, the kindergarten teacher informed his parents that he was playing in a disorganized and inconsistent manner. A more thorough psychological assessment, which was conducted during elementary school, indicated that Toby's level of intelligence is slightly below the average score (IQ = 93), but still within the normal range. Specific cognitive difficulties were observed in verbal comprehension, reading, and mathematics (standard scores ranged from 80–90). "Fortunately", according to the authors, Toby had a pleasant temperament and even if he fooled around at times, he had no behavioral problems. But, in 4th grade, it all began to unravel.

As school demands increased, Toby began to exhibit behaviors indicative of distraction and impulsivity, as well as oppositional and disruptive behaviors in the classroom. According to the authors, these behaviors appeared "because of a decline in academic performance" that happened during 5th grade (p. 318). Soon enough Toby received a diagnosis of ADHD and was prescribed with Lisdexamfetamine, an expensive and 'improved' stimulant medication known as Vyvanse. In the first few days, the medication led to an improvement in Toby's ability to concentrate (along with a decrease in appetite and difficulty falling asleep), but after a week, Toby started behaving strangely. He was anxious, picked at his lips, and chewed objects. His concentration abilities became abnormal. He was hyperfocused on just one activity, in a repetitive and relentless manner. For example, he would repeatedly draw the same objects, over and over again, across piles of pages. As a result, even when he wanted to play with other children, he was unable to disconnect from his compulsive behavior.

After three weeks, Toby's worried parents asked their doctor to stop the medication, but stopping it caused an unexpected deterioration. It seemed as if, all of a sudden, Toby's entire personality had changed. For three consecutive days, Toby was exceptionally energetic, irritable, and angry. He began to behave in an uncharacteristic way, harassing other children and cursing. According to his parents, it looked like "ADHD on steroids". His parents rushed to get him the older, and more researched, medication (i.e., methylphenidate), but this medication did not yield positive outcomes, so they reverted to the original one.

After two months of stereotypic behaviors, during a school vacation, another attempt was made to stop the medication, but this time, Toby's reaction was severe. According to the authors, it was much beyond a plain recurrence of ADHD symptoms. Toby's behavior became hypersexual, hyper-hyperactive, provocative, and aggressive. When Toby returned to school, he began taking the medication again, but the compulsory behavior also returned, until his parents could no longer bear it and decided to stop the pharmacological treatment immediately.

In the third attempt to stop the medication, the problematic and inappropriate behaviors had become dangerous. Toby tried, for example, to jump out of a driving vehicle. He threw a bottle at a police officer, set fire to a store, destroyed his classmates' belongings, and exposed himself in public. These behaviors led to his hospitalization in a psychiatric institution, where Toby was diagnosed with acute mania and treated with anti-psychotic medications and mood stabilizers.

Fortunately, thanks to Toby's parents, the story did not become a tragedy (of a chronic psychiatric patient). Toby's parents sought a second opinion to find out if Toby was truly suffering from an acute bipolar disorder that had just surfaced. During this reevaluation, the second-opinion doctors determined that Toby's abnormal behaviors were essentially withdrawal manifestations — extreme reactions to the toxic medication for ADHD (a DNA testing ruled out the possibility that Toby's reaction to the medication was idiosyncratic). Essentially, in the authors' words, Toby experienced a "stimulant-induced mania" [2, p. 320].

All's (almost) well that ends well. Seven months after Toby's discharge from the hospital, all of his psychiatric medications were stopped, and the manic episodes had vanished completely. According to the authors, Toby is still a child who tends to hyperactivity and impulsivity, and his academic performance is still not good. However, his teachers manage to guide and supervise him, and he currently has many friends and hobbies [2].

Considering Toby's normative developmental history, along with his somewhat limited school-related cognitive abilities (e.g., in mathematics and reading tasks), Toby's case study is a powerful illustration why the information of this book cannot remain hidden from the public. Yes, Toby experienced some difficulties in school, but these difficulties are **not** manifestations of a neurodevelopmental disorder, but simply a reflection of his innate personality and skills, which are less compatible to mainstream educational settings. It seems that Toby became a victim of our societal tendency to medicalization [3]. Rather than addressing his challenges through psycho-educational means, Toby's teachers and doctors perceived them as a genuine pathology. They labeled the challenges with the most common neuropsychiatric label (ADHD) and chose to address them through the use of the most common medical treatment (stimulant medications). From that point, Toby's story escalated rapidly. The medications were not effective. On the contrary, they exacerbated his symptoms ("ADHD on steroids") and triggered serious psychiatric reactions. The original physician who prescribed the medication was reluctant to attribute these reactions to the medications and recommended of psychiatric hospitalization — a serious action, which triggered additional and more severe psychiatric labeling (a bipolar disorder) and more dangerous psychiatric interventions (Lithium).

Toby's story ended well, but the sharp-eyed reader must have noticed that I added one word to the Shakespearian phrase above: "All's well that ends well". Toby's personal story may have ended well, but it sheds light on many other cases in which worried and devoted parents trust the medical establishment, which does not hurry to share the information regarding the potential adverse outcomes of false psychiatric labels and regular stimulant use. Not all parents have the courage and the resourcefulness of Toby's parents — necessary assets that allowed them to confront the medical establishment and demand better care for their child. Many parents are accepting the prevailing biomedical position that perceives the amorphic label of ADHD as a concrete and real medical entity (see Chapter 1, for more information about 'diagnostic literalism'). They do not suspect that their doctors can prescribe medications that increase the risk for severe psychiatric reactions. Many of them might even believe their doctors when they insist that these reactions signify the existence of another pathology. The blame is of course, not on the coping parents, but on us, scientists and practitioners, who are not exposing the information about the fictitious 'illness' and about its dangerous 'cure', and who are not engaging in an uprising against the pressure inflicted on us by the pharmaceutical giants (Chapter 12). I can only hope that the consolidated information provided in this book would help us break free from the silencing influence of the illusory, biomedical consensus (Introduction).

The next section presents a mega table that might help us in this task, through a bird's eye view of the numerous validity gaps that tear down the biomedical consensus about ADHD (Table 4). In this section, which serves as a condensed representation of the entire scientific rebuttal, I also discuss the problematic reliance on non-parsimonious views (that are forced to implement multiple rationalizations and theoretical bandages) and I dare to draw the social and ethical picture that arises from this extremely large set of validity problems. Following this holistic rebuttal, I can finally propose key directions for short- and long-term change, based on the great literature that has accumulated on this topic.

A Time to Tear Down — 75 reasons why the biomedical consensus about ADHD is false

In order to prevent children from suffering, like the one described in Toby's story or the ones described in the stories of Billy, Oliver, and Elijah (Chapter 11), we have to tear down the consensual perception about ADHD. Table 4 provides an overview of the large collection of findings and facts documented in this book (N = 75) which undermine the various types of reliability and validity needed to maintain a solid scientific theory (i.e., for every finding/fact on the left column, the table indicates the major type of reliability/validity that is being impaired, using the warning icon ⚠). Notice that the validity terms that appear in the table are used in their broad meaning (see the technical **note** beneath the table, and the more elaborate description of the various types of reliability and validity brought in Chapter 1, **Box 1**). Following this mega table are a short philosophical discussion of the far-reaching implications of such a large collection of 'scientific holes', as well as a proposal for an alternative, and much more parsimonious, outlook on ADHD.

Table 4. A bird's eye view of the reliability and validity impairments in the biomedical consensus

	Findings and facts documented in this book	Reliability (stability)	Internal validity	Ecological validity	Construct validity
	Introduction: Illusory consensus and silenced controversy				
1	In contrast to conclusive statements, the scientific consensus is illusory. Multiple experts disagree with the ruling, biomedical theory regarding ADHD and its related medications.				⚠
Part One — ADHD is not an illness					
	Chapter 1: The philosophical foundation of the debate				
2	Despite the alleged neurobiological nature of ADHD, its clinical diagnosis relies on *subjective* measures like all other psychopathologies (readers should be careful of "diagnostic literalism").	⚠			⚠
	Chapter 2: The criterion of Deviance				
3	The prevalence of ADHD, according to the *DSM* (5%) is relatively high, considering the 2 standard deviation rule-of-thumb, and the prevalence of other childhood neurodevelopmental disorders mentioned in the *DSM*.				⚠
4	The prevalence of ADHD soared dramatically within 40 years, without a reasonable evolutionary explanation. Today, ADHD is an extremely common diagnosis (some studies evidenced over 20% rates).	⚠			⚠

(*Continued*)

Table 4. (*Continued*)

	Findings and facts documented in this book	Reliability (Stability)	Internal validity	Ecological validity	Construct validity
5	Many studies assess ADHD at the present moment, in a given cohort, despite the presumed biogenetic nature of the disorder, which implies that the prevalence of the diagnosis is accumulative.	⚠			
6	De facto, ADHD rates fluctuate significantly. ADHD does not "occur in most cultures in about 5%" as stated in the *DSM*, neither between countries, nor within countries.	⚠			⚠
7	ADHD rates depend on almost every sociodemographic parameter (e.g., gender, age, ethnicity).	⚠			⚠
8	Some cultural groups are more tolerant to ADHD-like behaviors, while others prefer to label them as a medical condition. Underprivileged children are being labeled more than others.	⚠			⚠
9	US Centers for Disease Control and Prevention rates suggest that for every single correct diagnosis (based on the *DSM* estimate), there are approximately two false ones. Most clinicians agree that ADHD is over-diagnosed, implying that the current definition of ADHD is problematic.	⚠			⚠
10	Despite the previous item, consensus members claim that ADHD is, in fact, under-diagnosed. Aside from the reliability problem, this claim suggests that ADHD rates are even higher than they are now.	⚠			⚠

	Chapter 3: The criterion of Dysfunction		
11	The entire list of ADHD symptoms in the *DSM* is based on the single criterion of dysfunction.		⚠
12	ADHD is an ever-changing concept (also, the contemporary formulation of ADHD, which focuses on 'attention', only emerged after the discovery of the cognitive effects of stimulants).	⚠	⚠
13	"Significant impairment" was softened to interference/reduction in functioning — a meaningless criterion that does not align with other neurodevelopmental disorders and with natural neurodiversity.	⚠	⚠
14	The phrasing of the symptoms reflects minor behavioral difficulties. The *DSM* allows a diagnosis of a "mild" disorder, which, by definition, does not meet the "Four Ds" criteria.		⚠
15	The word "often" that opens all 18 symptoms lacks a distinct cut-off point. There is no empirical evidence for "a discrete, nonarbitrary symptom severity threshold with regard to impairment".	⚠	
16	ADHD scales suffer from poor inter-raters' reliability: Teachers provide different ratings from parents and mothers provide different rating from fathers.	⚠	
17	There is a large overlap between the various symptoms of ADHD (a child who often runs about is also a child that is often unable to take part in quiet activities and often leaves seat).		⚠

(*Continued*)

Table 4. (*Continued*)

	Findings and facts documented in this book	Reliability (Stability)	Internal validity	Ecological validity	Construct validity
18	Dysfunctions mainly appear in school. The *DSM* provides multiple school-related examples, uses a softened '2-settings' requirement, and allows the absence of symptoms in other contexts.				⚠
19	ADHD children can sustain attention for prolonged periods and excel in tasks that require high cognitive control. This fact can even be seen in Computerized Performance Tests (CPTs), pending the removal of 'boring elements', thus suggesting that the main 'problem' is motivational, rather than purely cognitive.		⚠		⚠
20	The hyperfocus rationalization is not part of the symptomatology of the disorder. It is also not empirically proven and not in line with the theoretical definition of the disorder as: Attention Deficit.		⚠		⚠
21	In certain contexts, the characteristics of ADHD are actually strengths (e.g., creativity, high spirit, bravery).				⚠
22	The 'required' medications are used almost exclusively in school-related contexts. They are rarely used during vacations or for other purposes.				⚠
23	ADHD rates drop during adulthood. Multiple children do not meet the diagnostic criteria when they become adults. Cognitive functions, impulsivity, and hyperactivity improve naturally with age.	⚠			⚠

24	The dependency on age exists also within unified cohorts of children: ADHD and related treatments are more prevalent among children who are younger than the majority of their classmates.	⚠		⚠
	Chapter 4: The criterion of Danger			
25	The danger criterion is not manifested in the *DSM* list of symptoms.			⚠
26	ADHD does not cause premature death among children. Comorbid disorders and stimulant medications might do (see also Chapter 11). The mortality narrative is presented in a biased manner.		⚠	⚠
27	The small relationship between suicide risk and ADHD among adults is mediated by comorbid disorders and stimulant use.		⚠	⚠
28	Non-fatal serious dangers (e.g., incarcerations, car accidents), are irrelevant to children (the absolute risk is negligible). Medications in childhood (that work for several hours) were not proven to protect against future dangers (see also Chapter 9).		⚠	⚠
29	Much of the danger-related research is based on poor logic (A → B does not equal B → A), without evidence for direct causal relationships and without consideration of sociological factors.		⚠	
30	Risk-taking, which is associated with ADHD, is also associated with gender. Men take more risks than women. This does not mean they suffer psychopathology.			⚠

(*Continued*)

Table 4. (*Continued*)

	Findings and facts documented in this book	**Reliability (Stability)**	**Internal validity**	**Ecological validity**	**Construct validity**
31	Boys are consistently diagnosed and medically treated more than girls (rates are extremely high among adolescent males). It seems that plain gender differences are pathologized unjustifiably.	⚠	⚠		⚠
32	Female caregivers are inclined to identify boys with ADHD more than males. Differences in the number of prescriptions can be explained through differences between school staff.	⚠	⚠		⚠
33	Some presentations of ADHD do not share even one common symptom (an energetic and noisy boy suffers from the same brain deficit as the quiet dreamy girl, and both receive the same treatment of choice).				⚠
34	Risk-taking can be rewarding. ADHD-related characteristics can be seen as an evolutionary advantage (e.g., the gorilla study) that could be leveraged in life (e.g., entrepreneurship).				⚠
35	There are numerous examples of ADHD children who grew up to be functioning and even successful adults. Many of them are proud of their diagnosis and will not trade it.				⚠

	Chapter 5: The criterion of Distress		
36	The distress component in ADHD cannot be separated from adverse school experiences. Studies essentially investigate children who struggle with sitting and concentrating, the very behaviors that are demanded in school. The distress seems to result from a third variable. Children with high sensation-seeking needs (mostly boys) suffer in boring lessons (remember the electrifying study published in *Science*).	⚠	⚠
37	Consumer behaviors regarding the medications suggest that the clinical significance of ADHD-related distress outside of school context is minimal.		⚠
38	The distress component does not appear in the *DSM* criteria. ADHD is an example of the *DSM* guiding rule not to give psychiatric labels to conflicts between individuals and societies/expectable responses to common stressors.		⚠
39	Differential diagnosis is extremely complex (16 alternative conditions in the *DSM*, compared to 3–7 possibilities in other neurodevelopmental disorders). Multiple medical and other life conditions can trigger ADHD-like symptoms. Severe clinical cases that do meet the Four Ds criteria (Figure 2) are probably not ADHD (also because the severe symptoms are not part of the diagnostic criteria of the disorder). If we wish to preserve the label of ADHD to describe the small percent of highly disturbed children, we have to reconceptualize the disorder and update its diagnostic criteria.		⚠

(*Continued*)

Table 4. (*Continued*)

	Findings and facts documented in this book	Reliability (Stability)	Internal validity	Ecological validity	Construct validity
40	Most children with severe ADHD (70–80%) have at least one additional comorbid disorder. The efforts to create (intimidating) convergent validity eliminated the prerequisite for discriminant validity. Moreover, even small numbers of serious pathology that is not ADHD bias experimental results.		⚠		⚠
41	The prejudice and negative stigma that are typically associated with mental disorders seem to disappear in ADHD.				⚠
	Chapter 6: The neurobiology of ADHD				
42	Like all other psychopathologies, ADHD is not detected or diagnosed clinically through objective physiological measures, such as neuroimaging tools or other biological tests.				⚠
43	The reliability and validity (predictive, content, and ecological validities) of Computer-based Continuous Performance Tests (CPTs) are extremely poor.	⚠	⚠	⚠	
44	Decades of neurobiological research had never translated into objective and valid diagnostic measures in the clinical field.			⚠	
45	The very existence of brain differences is not enough to indicate the existence of a psychiatric condition and much of the research is "small in size and statistical power".		⚠		⚠

46	Mega-analyses yielded evidence that brain differences in childhood vanish in adulthood. In contrast to the neurobiological theory, the differences (in childhood) were not evident in the continuous scale and their overall contribution (i.e., effect size) to the explained variance in ADHD was null.		⚠		⚠
47	Multiple neuroimaging studies did not consider the expected artifact effects of the medications (i.e., the observed brain differences could have been the result of prolonged medication use).		⚠		
48	A large meta-analysis of 96 neuroimaging studies showed that there is no significant brain regional convergence in ADHD (the replication requirement is not met).	⚠			⚠
49	The selective/paradoxical effect of the medications is a myth: Medications cannot recognize where humans drew the dichotomous-diagnostic line (within continuous scales). Non-ADHD students abuse medications to enhance academic performance. Drug-induced (short-term) improvements do not depend on symptoms severity/existence of ADHD.		⚠	⚠	⚠
50	Contemporary mainstream psychiatrists renounce the "bogus chemical imbalance theory". Research on neurotransmitters yielded heterogenic results (including null results). Multiple studies did not consider the effects of the medications, which impact neurotransmitter levels (Chapter 11).	⚠	⚠		⚠
51	A review of 14 years of research revealed that there are more studies that *did not* find genetic links to ADHD than studies that did, and that the latter were not replicated adequately.	⚠			⚠

(Continued)

Table 4. (*Continued*)

	Findings and facts documented in this book	Reliability (Stability)	Internal validity	Ecological validity	Construct validity
52	Both the above lines of research, on brain differences and on genetic differences in ADHD, suffer from a significant publication bias.		⚠		
<u>Part Two — Ritalin is not a cure</u>					
	Chapter 8: Short-term efficacy of stimulant medications				
53	A literature review and meta-analysis of 185 Randomized Control Trials (RCTs) by the Cochrane revealed that the short-term efficacy of the medications is minor and mostly school-related (as reported mainly by teachers).				⚠
54	The medications generally do not improve academic performance or quality of life, and people rarely use them for managing other aspects of life that are not school-related.				⚠
55	Even the minor short-term benefits are judged to be overestimated due to inherent biases, such as: teachers' reports, significant publication bias, and numerous additional distortions (Chapter 12).		⚠		
	Chapter 9: Long-term efficacy of stimulant medications				
56	There is very little, high-quality longitudinal research on ADHD medications. The lack of adequate research on long-term efficacy is admitted by proponents of the medications.		⚠		

57	The data that do exist (e.g., from the MTA study) suggest that the medications have zero long-term efficacy in symptom reduction, academic improvement, or other cognitive and emotional domains.				⚠
58	In fact, when used for prolonged periods, the medications seem to produce 'reverse efficacy', that is: to exacerbate ADHD-like symptoms, Oppositional Defiant Disorder (ODD) behaviors, and overall functioning impairments.				⚠
59	Medications were not proven to protect against (hypothetical) ADHD-related dangers. The limited available research yielded heterogeneous, null, and mainly biased findings. The leaflet of the Ritalin states that medication breaks during holidays are expected, thus challenging the 'protection' notion.	⚠	⚠		⚠
	Chapter 10: 'Non-serious' safety concerns of stimulant use				
60	Medication studies typically have high proportions of dropouts — participants who cannot complete the study because of the adverse effects of the experimented medication.		⚠		⚠
61	In contrast to consensual reassuring messages, stimulants have numerous and highly prevalent 'non-serious' outcomes (e.g., tics, emotional lability, sleep problems, and ADHD-related symptoms), of which many are fairly serious (e.g., growth suppression, anorexia, anxiety, and depression). Many children resist taking the medications and consensual bodies downplay and even ignore the well-documented adverse outcomes of the medications.		⚠		⚠

(Continued)

Table 4. (*Continued*)

	Findings and facts documented in this book	**Reliability (Stability)**	**Internal validity**	**Ecological validity**	**Construct validity**
62	The desirable calming effect of the medications is likely to be a misrepresentation of the well-documented adverse effects of lethargy, apathy, zombie-like behaviors, and depression.		⚠		⚠
63	The desirable improvement in attention following the administration of the medications might be a misrepresentation of the adverse effects of OCD-like cognitions and behaviors.		⚠		⚠
64	Taken together, the questionable validity of the disorder, the unproven efficacy of the medications, and their numerous adverse outcomes suggest that non-medical reasons are involved (perhaps to overpower children).		⚠		
	Chapter 11: Serious safety concerns of stimulant use				
65	There is evidence for increased risk of suicide following stimulant use. This concern is typically dismissed by consensus members and concealed in the consumer leaflet.		⚠		⚠
66	A large body of research provided evidence that stimulant medications increase the risk for cardiovascular problems. This concern seems to be shared also by consensual authorities.				⚠
67	Evidence from human and nonhuman primate studies suggests that, in some cases, there is a causal link between stimulant use and onset of psychosis/mania. This link is repeatedly misrepresented and rationalized through improbable justifications (e.g., a prodrome, preceding psychosis).		⚠		⚠

68	In contrast to the (unproven) conceptualization of ADHD as a brain/chemical imbalance disorder (Chapter 6), studies on humans and mice suggest that ADHD medications can actually trigger biochemical dysregulations and prolonged changes in the brain.		⚠
69	In contrast to reassuring messages, ADHD medications are addictive, whether physiologically, through compensatory mechanisms, which cause long-term changes in the dopaminergic system, or psychologically (e.g., through behavioral conditioning).		⚠
	Chapter 12: Biases and conflicts of interests		
70	The NIMH webpage on the MTA study ignores the available longitudinal unfavorable findings that emerged from the study throughout the years.	⚠	
71	Large money is involved. ADHD medications are best-sellers to parents, and pharmaceutical companies spend millions on 'presents' to physicians — presents which are proven to increase sales.	⚠	
72	Numerous studies/researchers in the field received direct or indirect funding from pharmaceutical companies. Conflicts of interest are not always adequately reported.	⚠	
73	Meta-analysis on the benefits of methylphenidate exposed a significant publication bias. This bias (together with publication biases from Chapters 6 and 8) is intensified by economic interests.	⚠	

(*Continued*)

Table 4. (*Continued*)

	Findings and facts documented in this book	Reliability (Stability)	Internal validity	Ecological validity	Construct validity
74	The majority of the 260 studies reviewed by the Cochrane were rated with very poor quality and critical risk of bias (see inside the chapter for a range of misconducts and biases). Not surprisingly, funded studies usually report fewer adverse outcomes of medications than non-funded studies.		⚠		
	General Discussion: A time to tear down				
75	Lack of scientific parsimony leads to instability of the theoretical structure (see next).				⚠

Note: An informative description of the various types of reliability and validity is available in Box 1 (Chapter 1). For every finding/fact on the left column, the current table indicates (through the warning icon ⚠) the major types of reliability/validity that are being impaired. In the spirit of this book, this table relates to the various reliability/validity terms in their broad meaning. Briefly, *reliability* refers to accuracy and stability of variables. The various types of reliability (e.g., inter-rater reliability) serve as a prerequisite condition for further validity. *Internal validity* refers to the scientific strength of a given research and its ability to rule out alternative explanations (RCTs for example are considered a gold standard, while poor-quality research and inherent biases impair our ability to derive valid conclusions). In this table, this type of validity is also used to describe the strength of a given argument within the theory (i.e., an argument that is not empirically or logically supported is classified as an argument with poor internal validity). *Ecological validly* refers to the generalizability of given findings to various contexts. *Construct validity* includes *convergent and discriminant* validity, which address the degree to which items form a unified (convergent) cluster that is clearly distinct (discriminated) from other clusters. Importantly, this type of validity (which is typically used in the field of psychological testing) is used in the current table also to describe the soundness of the overall organizing theory (i.e., the biomedical consensus about ADHD and stimulant medications). In other words, findings and facts that do not align with the theory are classified as indicators of poor construct validity. In a way, all types of reliability and validity problems might impair the theory's *construct validity*. A certain degree of overlap between the various types of reliability and validity is also expected because problems in one type of reliability/validity typically trigger further problems in other types.

A time to cast away (non-parsimonious theoretical) stones and redefine ADHD

ADHD experts representing the alleged consensus probably have an excellent excuse for each and every validity item presented in the mega table (Table 4). However, this is exactly the case where the auxiliary philosophical-scientific rule, known as the principle of parsimony [4], or "Occam's Razor", should be considered. When there are several possible explanations for the same phenomenon, scientists are recommended to use a metaphorical razor to cut complex explanations and prioritize frugal explanations that involve the least number of theoretical concepts and stipulations.

When the consensus members insist, almost dogmatically, that ADHD is a valid neuropsychiatric disorder, they ought to keep integrating more and more conceptualizations and rationalizations, desperate tennis swings if you will, aimed at rescuing the collapsing theoretical tower of ADHD. Some of these swings are so weak that even the most talented consensual players, backed by an army of scientists, and sponsored by large pharmaceutical companies, give up on substantive responses and switch to insults and accusations (for examples, see the Introduction and my Personal Prologue). Instead of confronting the 'logos' (the substance) of our critical arguments, they turn to direct assaults on their 'pathos' and 'ethos', that is, the emotional aspects of the arguments and the credibility of their messenger (e.g., you are just a Doctor of Philosophy, not a real Medical Doctor like we are). They might even call their opponents: "a handful of nonexpert doctors" that "publish stories" that tantamount to "declaring the earth flat, the laws of gravity debatable, and the periodic table in chemistry a fraud" [1].

Let them continue their attacks as they wish. The same cliché that works in football is relevant to tennis as well: The bird's eye table doesn't lie. There are at least 75 reasons why ADHD should not be included in the *DSM*. All we need is to zoom out from the list of 18 (overlapping and unreliable) *DSM* symptoms, which all relate to the softened (and practically meaningless) criterion of a reduction/interference in functioning, and ask a simple question: In what context are these mild symptoms expressed and where exactly are these symptoms likely to cause emotional distress? When this is done, it will be possible to come up with a parsimonious response to the long list of validity deficiencies presented in the mega table. It is true. Children differ from one another. Neurological diversity dictates that some children will be more energetic and more distracted than others. However, this diversity does not mean that they have a neuropsychiatric disorder. There is no need to add superfluous conceptualizations such as "brain defect" (which apparently cannot be seen in neuroimaging studies), a "chemical imbalance" (a myth that originates from a false hypothesis regarding the selective/paradoxical effects of the medications), or extreme comorbidity (which eliminates our ability to distinguish ADHD from other conditions).

A much more parsimonious response would return to the null hypothesis (H0), according to which *all children are normal until proven otherwise* and raise the simple hypothesis that the concept of ADHD essentially reflects *a tragic encounter between normative traits of numerous children and their educational surroundings*. The more the school demands of dreamy or energetic children 'to behave nicely' and pay attention to boring teacher-fronted lessons, the more the prevalence, the dysfunctions, and the distress that are associated with the phenomenon called ADHD will increase. As shown multiple times in this book, school settings are the place where the Dysfunction and Distress components of ADHD are most evident (the other two "Ds" are usually not met, even in the context of school). This is because energetic/daydreaming children who have a hard time sitting and concentrating are requested to do these very things: To sit and focus, lesson after lesson, six days a week, for at least 12 years. No wonder, they feel distressed. In a way, these children are like a homosexual adolescent who grows up in a society that demands of him: Be straight! Be a man, try to make it with the girls. Be like everyone else.

Of course, ADHD-related behaviors can be quite annoying, but they are not pathological, and they are usually part of a multifaceted personality package that has, like all other human qualities, both advantages and disadvantages — distractibility and impulsivity on the one hand; openness, courage, curiosity, and creativity on the other. Now, we have two possibilities. One is to embrace this wonderful bundle of personality traits — let the child work on his roar, and see how he becomes a mighty lion king (like no king was before). The other is to regiment and engineer the child's behaviors by all kinds of peculiar methods so that he/she will fit into our old-school educational system. The only problem with this last option is that when you mix such a personality package with two liters of history or trigonometry and bake the resultant mix in a heated educational oven from 8.00 a.m. in the morning to 4.00 p.m. in the afternoon, the glass baking pan is bound to explode.

And no. Prescribing stimulant medications would not prevent this explosion. The medications cannot soften the sharp edges of this rough intersection between the child and the school. They might mask the real socioeducational problem for a short period of time, but after a while, they only make things worse. In my view, this common medical practice, which utilizes stimulant medications to fit ADHD-type children into a one-size-fits-all school, is not really different from the uncommon and highly condemned practice, in which ultra-religious institutions use psychiatric drugs to suppress their adolescent students' emerging sexuality. If stimulant medications were being given only to the very small percentage of children described in Chapter 5 (Figure 2), who suffer extreme distress and dysfunction — the small subgroup of children who are accidently labeled with ADHD despite their eligibility for a significantly more serious condition — I would probably not have felt the urge to write this entire book. But the current situation is unbearable. Parents are led to believe that ADHD is a highly dangerous condition, and stimulant medications are prescribed to children as if they were treats during Halloween. To me, the current situation starts to resemble the dystopic world created by Stanislaw Lem, the science fiction author of *The Futurological Congress* [5]. I would not be surprised if, someday, in the near future, students will learn about the bewildering era in history during which adults gave children psychoactive substances to control their behaviors and enhance their academic performance.

A Time to Build – 4 directions for change

But if ADHD is not an illness, and Ritalin not a cure, then what should we do to stop this dystopic tale and bring hope to our children? Great intellectuals have addressed this socioeducational question, and the current book does not have the mandate to provide comprehensive and detailed solutions to the continuous friction that characterizes the intersection between energetic/dreamy children and mainstream schools. However, with your permission, I do wish to outline **three** practical (though not easy) directions for change that can help the children of today thrive, despite the discouraging medical label, along with **one** conceptual, long-term direction that could help "the children of tomorrow dream away", as beautifully phrased by the scorpions.

A time to love (the children of today)

Balanced Parenting. The first principal solution concerns our very own approach as parents. Children with ADHD-like characteristics are typically not easy to raise. I am the first to admit this fact (see my Personal Prologue). This does not mean that these children should be medicated. Not at all. It only means that we need to work harder to (1) be a good *role model* for our children, (2) be *present*, and (3) adopt a compassionate, yet authoritative parenting style. Such a parenting style may not be intuitive to all parents, as many of us tend to be either too authoritarian (i.e., highly demanding and less sensitive) or too permissive [6]. However, since our children's emotional equilibrium depends on us, we have to find ways to provide them with unconditional love, without comprising on clear boundaries and proper discipline. If necessary, parents are advised (and I include myself in this group of advisees) to participate in a parenting class, in which we can strengthen our parental confidence and acquire practical tools that will allow us to discipline and educate our children on the one hand and increase their inner self-esteem and sense of worthiness on the other hand.

Instead of turning to dangerous psychiatric medications, let's be more present in our children's life and give them an overdose of love, understanding, and empowerment (and ourselves a hearty dose of patience and faith). It may sound like a naïve cliché, but I fervently believe that in most cases of so-called ADHD (i.e., not in the severe cases, which mask other, more serious conditions — see Chapter 5), a supportive and loving environment will allow the child's elastic brain to do what it does best during natural development, that is, to adapt and improve itself in the face of real-life changes and challenges [7, 8]. The mitigating effect of natural development on ADHD symptoms can be seen in the *spontaneous recovery* of most children (Chapter 3) and the positive course of the 'illness' in control groups of experimental designs, such as the one implied in the MTA study (Chapter 9). There is no logic, in my opinion, to gamble and provide still-developing children with stimulant medications that might impair their healthy developmental process (Chapters 10 and 11).

Non-pharmacological interventions. The second solution concerns the plentiful non-pharmacological interventions that are now available to what the consensus calls ADHD. Even if one accepts Barkley's conceptualization of ADHD as "the diabetes of psychiatry… a chronic disorder that has to be managed every day" (Introduction), this daily management does not have to include ineffective and unsafe medications. After all, Barkley himself admitted that "**there is no cure for this disorder**" (Introduction) and even chronic, type 2 diabetes might be managed regularly using non-pharmacological lifestyle accommodations (e.g., diet and exercise).

Although I call to stop relating to ADHD as a medical illness, I acknowledge parents' need for practical solutions and I advocate the integration of evidence-based non-pharmacological therapeutic interventions that can improve the child's cognitive and behavioral abilities (the child does not need to have a diagnosis to enjoy the benefits of non-pharmacological interventions). Such non-pharmacological interventions make use of diverse therapeutic approaches, including behavioral treatments [9], regular exercise [10], nutritional and environmental modifications [11], mindfulness therapies [12], and neurofeedback [13].

The scope of this book does not allow us to expand on each of the above non-pharmacological interventions, yet the last (i.e., the neurofeedback-based intervention) deserves a brief introduction because it is somewhat less prominent in the clinical field and it has a major potential to replace the use of the current treatment of choice [14] (don't worry, I do not receive funding for advocating this intervention). Historically, the use of neurofeedback is dated to only several years after the revelation of electroencephalography (EEG) — the popular brain monitoring method of electric activity. In neurofeedback-based therapy, patients receive real time feedback on their EEG activity, thus allowing them to identify the times their EEG exhibited the desired features associated with enhanced attention. This process trains the brain to more easily produce and maintain the brain activity pattern associated with enhanced attention [15].

Importantly for ADHD-type children, neurofeedback interventions can be administered through entertaining computer games, thus overcoming their tendency to get bored and facilitating their implicit learning of procedural skills at cognitive-control tasks that eventually become automatic (like riding a bicycle). Moreover, in line with the leading narrative of this book, the theory behind this type of intervention does not require that the child will be diagnosed with a medical illness. Neurofeedback is used also among healthy populations, as a straightforward cognitive enhancer tool, that utilizes the brain's natural plasticity to achieve positive outcomes without endangering its users. Specifically for ADHD, although the number of RCTs is still limited, a meta-analysis of the accumulating evidence suggests that neurofeedback interventions have sustainable medium-to-large positive effects, both right after treatment and during a longitudinal follow-up several months later [13].

The main limitation of neurofeedback interventions is their inherent requirement for specific equipment and trained operators. Readers should therefore know that there is a wealth of additional, relatively simple to administer, non-pharmacological techniques, which could bring an immediate relief [for fascinating examples, see in: 16, 17, 18]. Personally, whenever parents contact me for advice, I tend to utilize the comprehensive collection of non-medical interventions proposed by Dr. Thomas Armstrong, the prominent critic of ADHD mentioned in the Introduction. In the new edition of his book, Armstrong suggests no less than **101** non-pharmacological practical strategies, which can improve children's quality of life significantly [19].

To increase children's *cognitive abilities*, parents may teach their children organizational, cognitive functions, and learning strategies (strategies 7, 37, 51, 72, and 101), provide them with stimulating learning activities, perhaps through movement (strategies 50 and 56), and make use of screen-based technologies, such as learning apps and video games (strategies 40, 47, 83, and 84). To improve children's *resilience and emotion regulation*, parents may encourage marital arts and nature-based activities (strategies 4 and 5), utilize calming music, meditation exercises, and yoga (strategies 16, 43, and 87), and teach self-regulation and stress management skills (strategies 42 and 46). Finally, to improve children's inner *sense of independence and responsibility*, parents may appoint their children to be in charge of real-life tasks at home, take care of a pet, and be a big-brother mentor to a younger child (strategies 73, 81, and 88).

Parents, of course, do not need to apply so many strategies. The aforementioned strategies are presented here only to illustrate the richness and the availability of the non-medical possibilities (and because these are the strategies that I, personally, like the most). After all, if we wish to teach a child to be more attentive, have more patience and grit, and be less impulsive and disruptive, there is no logic to turn to medications. These are straightforward psycho-educational challenges that should be addressed through psycho-educational and parental measures.

Alternative education. The third, and more comprehensive direction concerns the child's school environment. Assuming that much of the child's difficulties arise in mainstream school context, parents may consider non-conventional learning environments, such as the emerging democratic-oriented schools [20]. Although different educational streams emphasize different values, most non-conventional schools typically apply a less dogmatic pedagogical approach, which prioritizes small-size classes, warm relationships between teachers and students, diverse educational experiences that involve movement and play, and strong focus on the child's unique strengths, fields of interests, and inner socioemotional world (over plain academic performance). These alternative streams typically nurture children's natural curiosity and strive for responsibility and independence, thus allowing them to acquire valuable real-life skills in a supportive and less judgmental environment that suits their unique needs and developmental stage [20–22].

Of course, not all children live next to such progressive educational institutions, and not all parents can afford their fees. However, I am not sure that the alternative option, that is, the choice to send sensitive ADHD-type children to mainstream schools, which will continue to bomb them with demands, reprimands, psychiatric labels, and dangerous drugs, is cheaper in the long run. Ritalin, we have to admit, is the poor solution of the poor. Whereas high socioeconomical strata may afford alternative pedagogical approaches and expensive non-medical treatments, parents who are less fortunate have less leeway, and in many cases, their life circumstances force them to give their children medications. This inherent discrimination brings us to the last, and most important conceptual direction for change, for which I wish to dedicate a separate heading.

A time to heal (the children of tomorrow)

Heal our daily language. Ostensibly, this book deals with semantic distinctions — "trait" or "mode of thought" instead of "disorder" or "illness"; "dangerous" or "ineffective" drugs instead of "medicine" or "cure" — but, if we manage to rectify the semantics, we will obligate the educational and the health systems to recalculate their routes and policies. Luckily, we have a precedent. In 1973, the American Psychiatric Association (APA) made an historical decision to *depathologize* homosexuality and remove this diagnosis from the *DSM* [23]. Today, this decision sounds trivial, but back in the 1970s, it probably shocked the believers of the diagnosis. I am aware that some people still hold negative attitudes towards the LGBT community, but the mainstream psychiatric-medical establishment denounces anyone who argues that homosexuality is a psychiatric disorder and condemns practitioners who 'treat' homosexuality with psychiatric drugs within the pseudoscientific framework of *conversion therapy*. Even those who insist that differences exist between the homosexual brain and the heterosexual brain acknowledge that homosexuality does not meet the "Four Ds" criteria of psychiatric diagnosis.

Now comes the turn of ADHD. Like homosexuality, ADHD also fails to meet the "Four Ds" criteria, certainly when we keep a distance between the pure 'mode of thought' and the external demands of the educational system. Very few parents give their child stimulants during weekends or summer breaks. Indeed, during the long summer vacation, the child can be "pretty annoying and loud". He probably "needs to be kept busy, otherwise he would drive his sister mad", but somehow, during the summer break, he's not sick. He doesn't need to take medications. Only when the new school year begins does he become sick again. It is a seasonal illness. It is therefore our duty to heal our daily language. Instead of falsely relating to ADHD as an objective innate brain disorder, we should remind ourselves, that like all human qualities, ADHD-type personality/mode-of-thought has both weaknesses and strengths, and that our role is to guide our children to cope with the former, and discover and realize the latter [24]. Once this insight is internalized, it will be much easier for us, as a society, to redefine the educational goals we wish to set for our children.

Heal our educational system. Indeed, powerful organizations are expected to resist this stormy wind of change, but we cannot let them intimidate us. It is our duty to take action. After all, as the popular meme says: "You can pray all you want, but eventually David had to pick up a stone and act against Goliath." Instead of allowing others to determine for us which child is worthy, and which child should be labeled with psychiatric diagnosis, let's change our educational beliefs. The existing educational model is based primarily on linguistic-verbal intelligence and logical-mathematical intelligence, while many ADHD-type children are blessed with other types of intelligences, such as naturalistic intelligence or bodily-kinesthetic intelligence [25]. Some of the diagnosed individuals, and especially those who were awarded the letter H, the honorary degree of Hyperactivity, are also characterized by a personal charisma, entrepreneurship tendency, creativity, and even leadership abilities (Chapters 4 and 5). It is therefore my belief that we ought to stop ranking children based on academic skills solely and start implementing insights from Gardner's inspiring *theory of multiple intelligences* [25]. There is no reason for our children to internalize a discouraging message as if a college professor is superior to a garage manager, a start-up entrepreneur, or a riding instructor on a horse ranch.

Except for cases of serious developmental deficits, such as Intellectual Disability or low-functioning Autism (see Chapters 1 and 5), the educational starting point should be that children have variegated abilities and personality traits. One might be shy and mathematically talented, and another might have difficulties with verbal-based subjects but is energetic and a social leader. Educational success, then, cannot be measured any more according to the percentage of students who go on to study at Ivy League colleges. That is because there is no single model of a proper educational product that fits all children. Along with the crucial need to reduce the number of children in the classroom and hire high quality teachers [26], policy makers are recommended to integrate diverged experiential activities that will match the multiple types of intelligence and personality traits of children. Regardless of ADHD, schools should also transform and adapt to the digital age [27] — the age of internet communication and screen technologies — which has a significant influence on how the children of today consume information, learn about the world, interact with their friends, and spend their leisure time [28].

The time has come to promote personalized education approaches [29] and create "the schools our children need" [26]. The theoretical knowledge is already out there. We can apply improved learning techniques from the field of *special-needs education*, which comprises a variety of accommodations to the inherent interpersonal variations that exist between children, and we can adopt the exciting approach and sophisticated equipment from the successful educational programs tailored for *gifted and talented children*. Indeed, these two special-education approaches require large financial investments, as they usually incorporate small classes, larger and highly trained teaching staffs, and expensive learning aids, but this investment will prevent further spending on medical and paramedical services for the many children who struggle with the current system.

This is all very nice (not to say naïve), but where would the money come from, for such a pervasive (not to say grandiose) change? From a practical, though somewhat revolutionary, point of view, I suggest that, at the beginning of this required healing process, the financial investments needed to improve our educational system would come at the expense of investments in pure academic achievements (unless governments can fund both). This might sound like heresy to some educators, but I propose that schooling will include less (but more quality) hours of formal learning than it does today, and more hours of social interactions and free play (within school premises and under light supervision of adult caregivers). Play has an essential role in healthy development [30] and, as such, it should be viewed as an integral part of good educational practice. Play contributes significantly to the child's cognitive and socioemotional functioning [31] and may prepare her/him for the unexpected and challenging events of the future [32]. The children of tomorrow may even like going to school, if play time is increased — a scenario that sounds like science fiction today. But think about it. Why do we accept this fact that so many children hate going to school? Indeed, we too suffered when we were children, but why do we perpetuate this bizarre custom? Of course, public schooling is essential for a functioning society, but it is time we improve it, so we can minimize the suffering of children, accommodate most types of children, and avoid the numerous casualties — the widespread neurodevelopmental labeling and the extensive drugging of millions of children.

A time to make history

I am actually quite optimistic. I have a strong, though not scientifically founded, belief that we are currently standing at a historical turning point. Until now, the ever-increasing rates of diagnoses and psychoactive treatments have taken place behind closed curtains. However, the diagnostic flood of the past years has crossed any reasonable barrier of *deviance* and the curtain seems to have begun rising, revealing an intuitive truth. ADHD has become "a national disaster of dangerous proportions", as openly declared by Dr. Keith Conners, the founding father of ADHD (Introduction), "a concoction to justify the giving out of medication at unprecedented and unjustifiable levels" [33]. Of course, not all scientists and doctors accept the position voiced in this book, but, in my opinion, they should at least inform the public about the controversy regarding the diagnosis and treatment of ADHD. Plain medical ethics require that.

The biomedical consensus, which has been perpetuated by the pharmaceutical companies in a self-amplifying echo chamber, is cracking. The over-prescription of stimulant medications is now flooding this consensual chamber, and scholars from all over the world are openly renouncing the biomedical paradigm. Of course, these scholars are not the majority yet; however, as mentioned in the Interim Summary of Part One, size should not matter in scientific discourse. The scientific consensus is always in consensus until it is not, as we all learned from the case of Galileo Galilei who was silenced by the scientific consensus of his time (the sacred Roman Inquisition). 'Real science', as termed by CHADD (Chapter 1), actually always leaves room for questions, criticisms, and debates, and the benefit of the doubt is typically reserved for the non-consensual scientists who dare to challenge the ruling theory. In fact, the burden of proof — the obligation to prove the validity of the scientific consensus — is imposed on the party that advocates it.

At this historical point, one might still try to paste more and more non-parsimonious bandages, in a desperate effort to hide the numerous scientific holes in the theoretical balloon, according to which tens of millions of children suffer from an incurable lifelong neuropsychiatric disorder. Alternatively, one can utilize the comprehensive rebuttal of the current book to pierce this over-blown theoretical balloon and join its call to remove the label of ADHD from the *DSM* altogether. As shown in this chapter, there are at least 75 reasons why the biomedical consensus is invalid, and I believe that real historical change is in our hands. As long as we do not cave, I dare to predict that the theoretical construct known as ADHD will eventually explode in the face of the charismatic and cheerful girl, or the bold and adventurous boy, who do not have any medical condition that meets the basic criteria of psychiatric diagnosis.

Now that we know that nothing is wrong with their brains, we can decide to embrace their complete and wonderful personality as it is, including their fidgeting, abounding energy, and uncontained joy and life force. We have the opportunity to establish, for these children, and for future generations, an education system that truly puts the well-being of the child at the center — even if he (or she) is having difficulties paying attention to the teacher, and prefers, instead, to dedicate his full attention to the removal of the stubborn gum that has been stuck under his table since last year.

Let's make history and build educational environments that are for, and not against, children — schools that accept the null hypothesis that all children are normal, unless proven otherwise.

References

1. Barkley, R.A., *International consensus statement on ADHD.* Journal of the American Academy of Child and Adolescent Psychiatry, 2002. **41**(12): p. 1389.
2. Friedland, S., *et al.*, *Stimulant-Induced Punding and Stimulant Discontinuation-Induced Manic-Like Symptoms in a Preadolescent Male.* Journal of Child and Adolescent Psychopharmacology, 2019. **29**(4): p. 318–320.
3. Maturo, A., *The medicalization of education: ADHD, human enhancement and academic performance.* Italian Journal of Sociology of Education, 2013. **5**(3).
4. Epstein, R., *The principle of parsimony and some applications in psychology.* The Journal of Mind and Behavior, 1984: p. 119–130.
5. Lem, S., *The Futurological Congress (from the Memoirs of Ijon Tichy).* 1985: Houghton Mifflin Harcourt.
6. Buri, J.R., *Parental authority questionnaire.* Journal of Personality Assessment, 1991. **57**(1): p. 110–119.
7. Doidge, N., *The brain that changes itself: Stories of personal triumph from the frontiers of brain science.* 2007: Penguin.
8. Rubin, B.P., *Changing brains: The emergence of the field of adult neurogenesis.* BioSocieties, 2009. **4**(4): p. 407–424.
9. Fabiano, G.A., *et al.*, *A meta-analysis of behavioral treatments for attention-deficit/hyperactivity disorder.* Clinical Psychology Review, 2009. **29**(2): p. 129–140.

10. Ng, Q.X., *et al.*, *Managing childhood and adolescent attention-deficit/hyperactivity disorder (ADHD) with exercise: A systematic review.* Complementary Therapies in Medicine, 2017. **34**: p. 123–128.
11. Curtis, L.T. and K. Patel, *Nutritional and Environmental Approaches to Preventing and Treating Autism and Attention Deficit Hyperactivity Disorder (ADHD): A Review.* The Journal of Alternative and Complementary Medicine, 2008. **14**(1): p. 79–85.
12. Cairncross, M. and C.J. Miller, *The effectiveness of mindfulness-based therapies for ADHD: a meta-analytic review.* Journal of Attention Disorders, 2020. **24**(5): p. 627–643.
13. Van Doren, J., *et al.*, *Sustained effects of neurofeedback in ADHD: a systematic review and meta-analysis.* European Child & Adolescent Psychiatry, 2019. **28**(3): p. 293–305.
14. González-Castro, P., *et al.*, *Efficacy of neurofeedback versus pharmacological support in subjects with ADHD.* Applied Psychophysiology and Biofeedback, 2016. **41**(1): p. 17–25.
15. Enriquez-Geppert, S., *et al.*, *Neurofeedback as a treatment intervention in ADHD: Current evidence and practice.* Current Psychiatry Reports, 2019. **21**(6): p. 1–7.
16. Hartmann, T., *Living with ADHD: Simple Exercises to Change Your Daily Life.* 2020: Simon and Schuster.
17. Timimi, S., *"I am struggling to cope with my child's behaviour and I think he may have ADHD": A brief overview of things to consider before going down the route of specialist services.* Journal of Childhood & Developmental Disorders, 2015. **1**(1): p. 5.
18. Timimi, S., *Non-diagnostic based approaches to helping children who could be labelled ADHD and their families.* International Journal of Qualitative Studies on Health and Well-Being, 2017. **12**(sup1): p. 1298270.
19. Armstrong, T., *The Myth of the ADHD Child, Revised Edition: 101 Ways to Improve Your Child's Behavior and Attention Span Without Drugs, Labels, or Coercion.* 2017: Penguin.
20. Sant, E., *Democratic education: A theoretical review (2006–2017).* Review of Educational Research, 2019. **89**(5): p. 655–696.

21. Easton, F., *Educating the Whole Child,"Head, Heart, and Hands": Learning from the Waldorf Experience.* Theory Into Practice, 1997. **36**(2): p. 87–94.
22. Marshall, C., *Montessori education: a review of the evidence base.* NPJ Science of Learning, 2017. **2**(1): p. 1–9.
23. Drescher, J., *Out of DSM: Depathologizing Homosexuality.* Behavioral Sciences (Basel, Switzerland), 2015. **5**(4): p. 565–575.
24. Poole, J., *Flipping ADHD on Its Head: How to Turn Your Child's "Disability" into Their Greatest Strength.* 2020: Greenleaf Book Group.
25. Gardner, H.E., *Frames of mind: The theory of multiple intelligences.* 2011: Hachette Uk.
26. Wiliam, D., *Creating the schools our children need.* 2018: Learning Sciences International.
27. Carlsson, H. and O. Sundin, *Searching for delegated knowledge in elementary schools.* Information Research, 2017. **22**(1).
28. Ophir, Y., *et al.*, *"Digital adolescence": The effects of smartphones and social networking technologies on adolescents' well-being,* in *Online Peer Engagement in Adolescence.* 2020, Routledge. p. 122–139.
29. Reber, R., E.A. Canning, and J.M. Harackiewicz, *Personalized education to increase interest.* Current Directions in Psychological Science, 2018. **27**(6): p. 449–454.
30. Almon, J., *The vital role of play in early childhood education.* All work and no play...How educational reforms are harming our preschoolers, 2003: p. 17–42.
31. Ginsburg, K.R., C. and the Committee on, and H. and the Committee on Psychosocial Aspects of Child and Family, *The Importance of Play in Promoting Healthy Child Development and Maintaining Strong Parent-Child Bonds.* Pediatrics, 2007. **119**(1): p. 182–191.
32. Spinka, M., R.C. Newberry, and M. Bekoff, *Mammalian play: training for the unexpected.* The Quarterly Review of Biology, 2001. **76**(2): p. 141–168.
33. Schwarz, A., *The selling of attention deficit disorder.* 2013, New York Times, Last retrieved in August, 2021 from: https://www.nytimes.com/2013/12/15/health/the-selling-of-attention-deficit-disorder.html.

Personal Epilogue
A very special flamingo

Upon completion of this book, it is time to admit that "long I stood" before I took the grassy road against the biomedical consensus. I already had the feeling ten years ago that something doesn't add up, when I witnessed the surprising recovery of Queen Sarabi's son (Personal Prologue), but I only started listening to winds of change a couple of years later, when my own first-born son, Maayan, was diagnosed with Attention Deficit Hyperactivity Disorder (ADHD). I remember vividly the time and place I decided to take this rocky road. It happened, exactly as the Scorpions' song predicted, "on an august summer night", in the magical Biblical Zoo of Jerusalem. My children and I arrived at the flamingos' ranch and there they were — proud, pink-colored flamingos, alongside majestic, white-colored flamingos, strolling around the field like prom queens, displaying their effortless, one-legged pose to all mankind.

Suddenly, Maayan noticed that one flamingo looked a bit different from the others. It was not exactly pink and not exactly white. It had instead a striped skin, which distinguished it from its flamingo friends. "Aba," he asked me with curious sparkling eyes, "why is this flamingo different from its classmates?" I shivered. Like most other questions my son had back then, when he was 4 years old, I did not know the answer to this one, but this question sounded as if it had a deeper, hidden meaning. I had to stall for time, so I pulled the oldest trick in my psychology book and responded with a question of my own: "What do you think? How does this striped flamingo feel?" Maayan did not hesitate for a moment and shot a sharp answer that stunned me: "I think it feels very special. Perhaps it can even do a perfect cartwheel."

I have no regret for traveling this unconventional road, but I admit that I had to retell myself the flamingo story many times throughout the writing process of this book, to remember why I have entered this minefield to begin with. Many times, throughout the writing process, I was bothered by discouraging thoughts that I am fighting a losing battle, that schools will never change, and that pharmaceutical companies will never let go of easy profit. "The pharma industry operates like the mafia," I kept hearing Peter Gøtzsche's warning, requiring me to respond quietly, like in a secret code: "except that the mafia kills less people".

But the truth is that I had almost no choice. Once I opened the Pandora's Box of ADHD in public, there was no way back. Parents from all over my country called me for help, insisting that this was the first time they felt understood. But I couldn't really help them. "Our education system is inflexible," I used to apologize, "the medical establishment is too powerful." I did try to direct them to alternative schools and suggest non-medical interventions, but I knew that, in most cases, I am only putting a temporary bandage on a severe fracture — a pervasive socioeducational problem. Writing this book, with the slightest hope that it will hasten the wind of change, was the minimum I could do for these coping parents.

Dear parents, I recognize that this book is written mostly in formal academic language, but it is addressed, first and foremost, to you (see my Personal Prologue). I share your pain and challenges and understand firsthand the difficulty of the Ritalin dilemma. In my view, mothers and fathers to ADHD-type children, like us, are the heroes of this historical tragedy. Please know that the criticism that appears in this book, is by no means directed at you. I know all too well how hard it is to maneuver through hostile territory — between the demands of our workplaces and the demands of our outdated education system, where our mischievous children (whose attention span reflects a typical story on Instagram), are expected to sit and concentrate for long hours. I truly hope that the consolidated information presented in this book will empower you to stand up against the institutionalized organizations and say: enough is enough. It is about time we take the power back from the drug companies and the medical establishment and build futuristic educational environments where the children of tomorrow can dream away, and where the learning can occur in the magic of the moment.

Resistance will not be easy. That's for sure. Like all big changes, the tectonic change that is required here would probably trigger intense rage by organizations that are stronger than us in terms of power and resources. But we cannot stay silenced anymore. If these establishments (let's call them Scar) wish to keep accusing us of not understanding the real pain of ADHD, or that we do not have the proper credentials to speak against the (pseudo) biomedical consensus, let them do so. This anticipated avoidance of a substantive discussion would only demonstrate the weakness of their arguments since real scientific discourse embraces debate. This is how science advances, as well put by Karl Popper, "through a process of trial and error, of conjecture and refutation". Personally, I prepare myself for their expected attempt to undermine my credibility, using derogatory terms and fancy psychiatric labels (something in the vein of a narcissistic personality disorder with a touch of savior fantasy and a drop of delusional thinking). After all, this is our profession, to give a bombastic name to human behaviors of others, precisely as we do nowadays to energetic and dreamy children in schools. I've heard that these lively children are tagged with an extravagant lifelong brain disorder called Attention Deficit Hyperactivity Disorder.

Little do they know that ADHD is Not a Disorder, and that Ritalin is Not a Cure. Little did I know that a decade ago, before I met Queen Sarabi. I thank you, dear lioness mother, from the bottom of my heart, for helping me to see that our energetic, curious, and sparkling children are perfect just as they are. And I thank you Maayani, my dearest son, for teaching me that different doesn't mean pathological and for giving me strength to speak up like Andersen's child hero. You are right. The consensual Emperor "hasn't got anything on". He may still order his noblemen and research assistants to keep holding his non-existent train, but he can no longer hide the naked truth regarding ADHD and its first-line treatments.

So, I dedicate this first-born book to you, my first-born son, my very special flamingo. Go, spread your wings, find your own personal wind, and dream away. Please try not to pay attention to those discouraging noises calling you bad names and please remember that you can always share your dreams with me. I promise to always stay close.

I love you, and I believe in you,

Aba

Acknowledgements

As you can imagine, the writing of this unconventional book was not an easy mission emotionally (see my Personal Prologue and Epilogue), and I doubt I could have completed this mission without the continuous support I received from my colleagues, friends, and family. It is my honor and sacred obligation to acknowledge their contribution here.

First among equals, I wish to thank Professor Emeritus Richard Silberstein from the Brain Sciences Institute at Swinburne University, who agreed to serve as the tough and uncompromising scientific reviewer of this book, despite his pleasant and humble nature. Richard, the resultant, high-quality content of this book is your doing, and I can't thank you enough. Also, please forgive me for all my queries and deliberations throughout the writing process. I truly hope I did not take advantage of your kind heart.

I also wish to thank my advisor at the Technion, Prof. Roi Reichart — a cherished friend and mentor who has been looking out for me in the tangled forest of academia, since we first met almost a decade ago in the best coffee shop in Jerusalem. Thank you, Roi, for encouraging me to pursue my research interests, even when they come at a price. Please know that insights from our long-standing conversations on 'science, medicine, and ethics', have penetrated this book, despite your insistence that your expertise does not include Attention Deficit Hyperactivity Disorder (ADHD).

My warm gratitude extends to my close academic 'Chavruta': Dr. Hananel Rosenberg from Ariel University, my dearest 'big brother' in the academy who enjoys teasing me, while supporting my endeavors and giving me the feeling that my research is truly revolutionary; soon-to-be Dr. Refael Tikochinski from the Technion, my secret genius weapon and trusted comrade, whose sharp-eyed remarks improved the quality of this book, as well as of many of my writings; Dr. Yaniv Efrati from Bar-Ilan University, a generous and most welcoming friend who always has the best academic tips and tales; and Dr. Yaffa Shir-Raz, the medical-scientific partisan who exposes me to the hidden backyard of science and gives me strength to stand up to giants.

The list of scholars from my wider academic circle to whom I owe thanks is too long to be provided here, but it is important to me to mention: Prof. Christa Asterhan and Prof. Baruch Shcwarz, from the Hebrew University of Jerusalem, who guided my first steps in the twists and turns of the academic world; Prof. Yair Amichai-Hamburger from Reichman University, a role-model from whom I learned that pioneering scientific breakthroughs are bound to encounter resistance; and Dr. Yuliya Lipshits from the Hebrew University of Jerusalem, a reliable friend who is always willing to provide counsel and support. I thank you all for contributing to my academic development, thus allowing the creation of this book.

The seeds of the book were sown several years ago, in the Hebrew articles I have published in *Haaretz* — an influential Israeli newspaper and *Hebrew Psychology* — a key communication outlet for mental health professionals. I hold deep gratitude and respect for editors Neta Achituv (from Haaretz) and Michal Alperstein, Guy Zwirn, and Ori Ferster (from *Hebrew Psychology*) who were the first to open their publication doors to my nonconventional views about the topic of this book (Guy, thank you for not letting me breach the boundaries of good taste). In fact, the lengthy articles I published in *Hebrew Psychology* served as the cornerstone upon which I constructed the current book. Other Israeli media, which allowed me to communicate my scientific critique to the public are: Kan 11 TV; Tel-Aviv Radio; Radio 103; Reshet 13 TV; Bhol.co.il, and Kan Resht Bet. Indeed, not all of them accepted my position, but I thank them deeply for giving me voice, where silencing has become the common prerogative.

Throughout the book, I have integrated some phrases and themes from cultural masterpieces, including: "The Lion King" and "Mulan" by Walt Disney, "The Road Not Taken" by Robert Frost, "The Futurological Congress" by Stanislaw Lem, "The Emperor's New Clothes" by Hans Christian Andersen, "The Hitchhiker's Guide to the Galaxy" by Douglas Adams, "To Everything

There is a Season" by Kohelet (Ecclesiastes), and "Wind of Change" by the Scorpions. I also utilized the high-quality language services (for which I paid without external support) of Academic Language Experts — a highly recommended business and enjoyed the (non-paid) language support of Gideon Weisz, a wise and kind-hearted American psychologist who identified with my first writings on the topic and volunteered to translate some of them, while refusing to get any compensation for his valuable contribution. Thank you, Gideon, from the bottom of my heart.

A special thanks is extended to my dear friend, Roman Wyden — a talented film director and a great thinker who is devoted to the mental health of ADHD-type children. Together with his gifted wife, Tatiana, Roman initiated the 'ADHD is over' project in which he produces their eye-opening podcast and their revolutionary documentary film that target fundamental issues closely related to the topic of this book. Roman, I learned from you a lot and it is an honor for me to appear on your show.

This is the place to give thanks to *Ethical Human Psychology and Psychiatry* (EHPP), an exceptional peer-reviewed scientific journal that is dedicated to the ethical consequences of scientific misconduct and problematic practices that occur in the field of mental health. EHPP is a lighthouse in a relatively dark ocean of biased research, and I am so proud its editor, Prof. Jacqueline Sparks, appreciated and published my work on the topic of this book. Another, less formal, yet highly valuable publication venue, which I owe thanks to, is *Mad in America*. This non-profit online magazine is one of the few platforms that challenge the biomedical views and practices in current psychiatric care and promote conceptual change. Specifically, I wish to thank its founder Robert Whitaker, a rare investigative journalist and an influential author, who agreed to share some of his decades of experience with me and answer my frequent emails with utmost patience and generosity.

Multiple others provided me great comments and insights throughout the writing process, including Prof. Matthew Smith from University of Strathclyde, author of a key critical book on the history of ADHD; Haviv Rettig Gur, a talented journalist by day and a shy intellectual by night; and Guy Ben-Zvi, who spotted typographical errors like the fighter pilot he is. Other great scholars, with whom I had never spoken in person, inspired the writing of this book without their knowledge. The list of these scholars is long (many of them are cited inside the book), but there are a few that had such a tremendous impact on my thinking, to the point that I feel obligated to convey my appreciation and gratitude to their indirect contribution here. This list includes Prof. James Swanson, Prof. Sami Timimi, Dr. Thomas Armstrong, Dr. Peter Breggin, and Thom Hartmann (Thom, I am so honored you read the preprint version of the book and decided to give it your full endorsement. Thank you very much).

Finally, I give thanks and warm hugs to my family members: to my dear mother who supports my mission despite her everlasting motherly concern; to my beloved father, the reason I became an academic researcher and the inspiration for my scholarly vision; to my brothers and sister, who suffered from my long speeches and gave me the feeling that my sayings are life-changing (I don't care if you lied, it worked anyway); to the best grandparents in the world, my father- and mother-in-law who treat me like their own son and get excited whenever I upload a video or publish an article (Savta Tony, here is the heart icon I promised you ♡); to my sister-in-law, Tali Weisbrun, the brilliant graphic designer who created the cover of this book, and, of course, to her charming daughter who agreed to be the presenter of the about-to-explode balloon.

Last, and by no means least, I thank my stunning children who give me power to overcome all obstacles and my beautiful, super-smart, and super-kind wife. Rony, my love, my rock, thank you so much for pushing me to write this book and ensuring that I have everything I need to do so. Whether it is King David or not, I hope the author of the book of Psalms will not be upset that

I am stealing his famous phrase and attributing it to you. Rony, “even when I walk through the darkest valley, I am not afraid, for you are close beside me”. Without you, I would never have had the strength to fight our son’s battle, resist the enormous pressure exerted on us by the medical/educational establishment and write this comprehensive rebuttal book.

What’s mine is yours,

Yaakov

About the Author

Dr. Yaakov Ophir is a research associate at the Technion — Israel Institute of Technology. He received his PhD from the Hebrew University of Jerusalem and gained extensive experience in complex empirical research and scientific criticism. Dr. Ophir taught several courses at distinguished academic institutions and published over 20 peer-reviewed scientific articles to date (with a specific focus on psychological development in the digital age and Artificial Intelligence tools for early detection of psychopathology). In his multiple, less formal 'popular science' writings and radio/television interviews (mostly in Hebrew), he manages to 'translate' complicated scientific ideas into plain concepts, which are accessible and even attractive to large audiences. Dr. Ophir is also a licensed clinical psychologist with a specific expertise in child therapy, parent training, and family interventions. He works at the mental health center of Megilot, in which he also served as the director of the 'National Program for Children and Youth at risk'.

Notably, these two complementary aspects of Dr. Ophir's professional profile are woven wisely into the current book through its exhaustive scientific inquiry and its embedded, real-life clinical knowledge. His expertise in knowledge translation is also evident. Although most of the book is written in a rigid and careful manner in line with standard academic style (especially considering its controversial content), Dr. Ophir approached the writing process from a personal and highly committed perspective — an approach that is reflected in the intense dynamic, colorfulness, and livelihood of the book. He opens and ends the book with authentic personal messages that pierce right through the hearts of the readers.

Index

Index

www.ingramcontent.com/pod-product-compliance
Lightning Source LLC
Chambersburg PA
CBHW061624220326
41598CB00026BA/3863
* 9 7 8 9 8 1 1 2 5 4 1 3 0 *